*Rural
Health Care*

WILEY SERIES IN HEALTH SERVICES

Stephen J. Williams, Sc.D., Series Editor

Rural Health Care

Roger A. Rosenblatt, M.D., M.P.H.
Associate Professor and Director
Research Section
Department of Family Medicine
School of Medicine
University of Washington
Seattle, Washington

Ira S. Moscovice, Ph.D.
Associate Professor
Center for Health Services Research
School of Public Health
University of Minnesota
Minneapolis, Minnesota

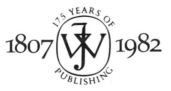

A WILEY MEDICAL PUBLICATION
JOHN WILEY & SONS
New York • Chichester • Brisbane • Toronto • Singapore

Library of Congress Cataloging in Publication Data:

Rosenblatt, Roger A.
  Rural health care.

  (Wiley series in health services, ISSN 0195-3907)
  Includes index.
  1. Rural health services—United States.
I. Moscovice, Ira S. II. Title. III. Series.
[DNLM: 1. Rural health. WA 390 R813r]
RA771.5.R67   362.1'0425   82-4892
ISBN 0-471-05419-4   AACR2

Printed in the United States of America

10 9 8 7 6 5 4 3 2 1

To Fernne and Sarah, who put up with us

The system works by interchange, by trading among the parts, by collaboration. Creatures accommodate to each other, move to one side to make room, live by rules. Without interliving, the place could never work. . . . Every living form is engaged, one way or another, in feeding other forms. There is a kind of mutual responsibility at work, holding all the parts together. . . .

Lewis Thomas
Notes of a Biology-Watcher—The Strangeness of Nature
New England Journal of Medicine
298:1455, June 29, 1978

Foreword

I read this manuscript from the vantage point of someone who has been interested in the problems of delivering health care in rural areas since his medical student days before World War II. Since then, I have had experience as a general practitioner in a rural village and been involved, from time to time, in developing, administering, and evaluating programs in this field. I found this book to be a most useful and thoroughgoing generic treatment of the subject.

The problem of making good quality and socially acceptable personal health services readily available to people in rural areas is worldwide and has long been recognized in the United States. Even in nations that have national health insurance and those that have national health services, it has been found that special arrangements must be made to provide adequate medical care resources in an accessible form in rural areas. It is, therefore, to be expected that in the United States, which has neither a national health service nor national health insurance, ready access to personal health services continues to be a serious problem for significant sections of our rural population.

For a long time now, and particularly in the last decade or more, various measures to correct this deficiency have been adopted in this country by rural people themselves and by other concerned parties, such as foundations and governments at local, state, and national levels. Yet it is not at all clear that satisfactory solutions have been definitively developed and implemented. In the past decade or so the assistance provided by governmental bodies and foundations for projects to solve this problem have begun to require the adoption of specific programmatic goals and particular methods of program organization and operation. The unique characteristics of rural areas, such as the lower density of population, combined with the fact that many such areas are poor, create inherent obstructions to the development of needed facilities and the recruitment and retention of professional personnel if reliance is to be placed only on the "free market" approach. The implementation of two major federal initiatives—Medicare and Medicaid—in the mid-1960s, while ameliorating somewhat the financial burden of medical care costs for the elderly and the very poor, served to highlight the special, continuing problems of rural people in obtaining access to care.

Clearly, there is no quick fix for this problem, and there is no single solution that will be suitable or feasible in all rural areas. Programs developed to solve this problem in the recent past on the American scene, in ways other than traditional solo practice, can be classified into four developmental strategies: the community health center, organized group practice, freestanding primary care centers, and institutional extension. A review by one of my colleagues, T. R. Konrad, of the types of social change that form the basis of the strategies that have been used, draws pertinent attention to theoretical issues fundamental to the achievement of the goal.

The individualistic theory focuses on the characteristics of the individual provider or other persons involved in the organization of the program with the idea that these people are viewed as change agents whose individual characteristics are thought to be critical ingredients to developing a successful enterprise. The institutional strategy is based on the thesis that social change comes about from the outside by the expansion of an established center leading to the incorporation of the periphery—the rural area—into an integrated system. The organizational design is a strategy of intervention that relies on the assumption that a particular kind of organization is the basic lever for the changes that are needed, thus placing the responsibility for success or failure of this type of program on its conformity to a specific organizational design—an investment in a concept based on the rational–technical theory of social change. The fourth major strategy of intervention is based on the belief that the community is the major locus for social change. It implies that the primary actors in the process of changing the health care scene are the community participants themselves and that the responsibility needs to be placed on their shoulders, thus requiring a systematic attempt to identify those communities that are ready for, or can be prepared for, the introduction of such a program. The critical ingredient is thought to be that activated communities—whose needs are articulated and supported by appropriate skills and knowledge—can design their own programs according to the level and character of their needs. These four strategies are not mutually exclusive, and some elements of the processes of each are evident in many of the organized efforts to deal with rural health care problems.

While the various efforts undertaken have made medical care more accessible in a good many rural communities, there remains a series of major policy concerns for which clearly established answers are sorely needed. Among these are such crucial questions as the effect of the nature of the community upon the outcomes of these programs in terms of access to care, their stability, and impact on health; how much and what kind of adaptation to community differences is needed; in what specific ways does the organizational form of a project affect its productivity and the outcomes mentioned earlier; how does the nature and degree of community involvement influence the conduct of the program and its specific outcome; how consequential is financial support for various purposes, and in what scale and for what duration; what factors influence productivity; what is the effect of various incentives; how can one best determine the subsidy gap as a function of the community setting, the scope of services given, and the available sources of payment; what are the factors influencing the stability of professional personnel in these programs; and how valid are the requirements set by sponsoring agencies? In the face of the mounting pressure for cost containment in medical care it is desirable, if not inevitable, that decisions be made in the context of access and scope of care and their association with improvement in health status. In terms of rural programs, this question is virtually untouched. Though there is no doubt that many of the programs that have been sponsored have done some good, in these times knowing this is really not enough. For all human services, mounting pressures all around us are being voiced in such terms as: how can we get the most good for the most people out of a certain level of expenditures? For people in rural areas, with the special problems that are inherent in rural life, this question is particularly poignant.

For those interested in understanding the issues in making health services available for rural people, this book provides an excellent foundation. It discusses the social and economic contexts of rural life, the implications that these have for health care, and the evolution of the crisis in rural health care. After documenting the present situation with regard to health resources and health status in rural America, the fundamental role of primary care and the special role of the rural hospital are appropriately highlighted. Attention is also given to emergency medical care and to other program components that present special problems in rural areas, such as mental health, care for the elderly, and dental care. The final chapter, entitled "Toward a Strategy for Improving Rural Health Care," sets forth the basic principles needing attention if an effective rural health care system is to be developed. These include the importance of planning on a local population base with emphasis on primary care, integrating local services with specialist services and other relevant health resources in the region, building two-way cooperative arrangements with other rural and urban communities in terms of the concept of regionalization, structuring the payment system to reward appropriate rural health services effectively, and applying these principles to the major components of the resource capacity and organizations that provide services, such as strong medical practices, the rural hospital, meaningful community involvement, and partnership with government.

For some time now we have needed an up-to-date, comprehensive review of the background and status of rural health care in the United States. This book does this well and also delineates the basic ingredients that will make for future progress. It will be useful to all who are interested in rural health care, from health professionals to community leaders and government representatives and officials at all levels.

Cecil G. Sheps, M.D., M.P.H.
Taylor Grandy Distinguished Professor of Social Medicine
School of Medicine and Health Services Research Center
University of North Carolina at Chapel Hill
Chapel Hill, North Carolina

Preface

Rural America is in a state of transition, shaped by powerful social, economic, and demographic forces. The health care system is undergoing rapid change, and the inevitable collision between rising expectations and insupportable costs will force a major restructuring of the way health services are provided. This book examines in detail the way rural Americans currently obtain health services and builds upon our understanding of the present system to look at some of the choices that will confront us in the near future with regard to rural health care.

This book is for people who are involved in health care delivery in rural areas and for those interested in improving the general organization of health care services in the United States. More than one-third of Americans live in nonmetropolitan areas, and one of our focuses has been on how to bring high quality and efficient health care services to this segment of American society. We have based this work on a detailed examination of the current components of the rural health care system and illustrate the ways in which local decision makers and health providers can evaluate these components to determine the future of health services in their communities.

The broad scope of topics we cover ranges from a historical overview of the way in which successive generations have obtained health care in rural America to an explanation of individual aspects of the rural health care system, such as rural hospitals or emergency health care. *Rural Health Care* can be used as a text for those wishing a comprehensive introduction to the field, or it can be used as a reference source for those with an interest in a specific area. The tables and figures are current and bring together data from diverse sources. We have tried to organize the text so that the information is available to both the reader requiring easy access to particular facts and to the less hurried reader who wishes to examine some of the perplexing difficulties involved in providing health services to remote or sparsely populated areas.

An enormous amount of work has been done in the field of rural health over the last 30 years. Much of this work has been the by-product of public and private investment in improving the quantity and quality of health services available to sparsely populated areas of America. We have attempted to synthesize the extensive literature about these experiments in health service delivery and to highlight the problems that remain now that this unprecedented cycle of public intervention has begun to ebb. As responsibility for social and health services devolves increasingly on private practitioners and local government, we hope that this book will assist those who are continuing the process of making health care available and affordable for the rural American public.

We would like to thank our colleagues whose incisive criticism, patience, and suggestions have enabled us to write this book. We would like to express special gratitude to the following people who reviewed portions of the manuscript, helping us to clarify our ideas and adding important data: Jack Bartleson, Sherman Cox, David Doth, Jay Greenberg, Don Madison, John Mayer, Bruce Perry, Ted Phillips, Cecil Sheps, Naomi Silverstone, and Cynthia Watts. Diane MacKenzie and Laura Larsson helped us obtain hard-to-find bibliographic materials; Nancy Jacobs, Donna Rosenthal, and Paulette Anderson typed portions of the manuscript; and Martha Reeves used the magic of the word processor to make the multiple revisions possible. Final thanks go to the chairmen of our respective departments, Dr. John Geyman and Dr. Stephen Shortell at the University of Washington and Dr. John Kralewski at the University of Minnesota, whose support and encouragement enabled us to complete this work.

This book owes its existence to the many rural physicians, nurses, hospital administrators, and residents who gave us insight into the trials and the triumphs of health care delivery in rural America. To the extent that this book becomes a tool in their hands, our work has been worthwhile.

Roger A. Rosenblatt
Ira S. Moscovice

Contents

Rural
Health Care

CHAPTER 1

Health Care and the Social Fabric of Rural America

Health care plays a significant part in all our lives. The average American interacts frequently with the health care system, that euphemism for the tenth of the national economy that is devoted to the production and distribution of services designed to maintain the health and relieve the illnesses of the American people. The average citizen sees a physician several times a year, purchases a bewildering array of useless nostrums and powerful medications, rents medical devices, negotiates for improved health insurance, and worries about the physical and mental well-being of his family. The pursuit of health occupies a considerable portion of our time and attention as we jog doggedly around the block or struggle with a child-proof drug container. Health care is such a pervasive part of our daily lives that it is difficult to begin a rational dissection of its dimensions.

During the twentieth century we have learned to control and prevent the major lethal infectious diseases. Through population-based interventions—the development of adequate water and waste-disposal systems, the introduction of mass immunizations, and major improvements in levels of nutrition and basic human services—we have relegated childhood death to the status of a random fluke. As we have been able to guarantee a minimum life span—barring automobile accidents or aberrations of cells—

1

attention has focused on achieving equity in the distribution of the real and symbolic correlates of health—doctors, hospitals, and the whole gamut of health services.

This book focuses on health care in rural America. Rural America has long been identified as one demographic segment of the nation that has traditionally lagged behind more densely populated regions in the acquisition of basic social services, including health care. A conference on rural health care in 1939 noted, "Even a superficial examination of the medical writings of the last one hundred years will indicate that there has been scarcely a time or a place, in western nations at least, when there have not been complaints of a lack of medical services in rural areas."[1] The subsequent 40 years has intensified the public commitment to improving access to medical services for all segments of society, and rural America has been a major focus of much of the remedial attention. Our intent in this volume is to illuminate the function of health care in the sustenance of rural society, illustrate the current deficiencies in the provision of appropriate and dependable health services, and suggest an approach to their improvement.

RURALITY: WHAT IS IT AND WHAT ROLE DOES IT PLAY IN AMERICAN LIFE?

The agrarian ideal permeates American cultural history. Thomas Jefferson extolled the virtues of a democracy built on the base of a nation of free land-holders and decried the pernicious influence of dense population clusters. The farm bloc has powerfully pursued agricultural interests, and support for the farmer is part of the political repertoire of most aspiring presidential candidates. Yet, until recently, rural areas have been places where people came from, places left behind in the quest for education, better jobs, and the excitement of the city.

Rurality remains a Platonic ideal; it resists quantification. Most people have a firm notion of what constitutes a rural setting. When it is analyzed, the core of this perception of rurality is the degree to which the natural environment is unaffected by humans. The essence of a rural setting is that it is undisturbed, that it remains in its natural form. Allied to this notion is a bucolic romanticization of the rural environment, decorated by tree and glade, graced with a cool breeze and delicate flowers. Yet when the romantic coloration is removed, the rural environments are those that remain unperturbed by human creations.

In contrast to the relative clarity of the concept of rurality is its identification for statistical purposes. The urban/rural categories create confusion by forcing an artificial dichotomy. The size of settlements and population density are continuous variables, and there is no a priori logical method of dividing the continuum at any particular point. Yet, in an attempt to distinguish those attributes that are unique to or predominant in rural America, we are forced to make distinctions for the purpose of meaningful comparison.

Every published work on rural health care begins with this definitional struggle. The classic census definition is confusing in its simplicity. By lumping into the rural category all those who dwell in "open country" or in towns with fewer than 2,500 people, the Census Bureau does identify a segment of the people who inhabit rural America. Yet the qualities of rural life—both ecological and psychological—would seem to apply with equal force in a small community of 4,000 people; certainly to consider such a town as "urban" assails the conventional understanding of that notion.

The division of the population into nonmetropolitan and metropolitan, and the creation of the *Standard Metropolitan Statistical Area (SMSA)*, recognizes the futility of arbitrary demographic classifications built solely on population size. Yet once again the dichotomous classification does not do justice to those at the interface. When does a small residential village in Connecticut become a suburb of Manhattan? And since the SMSA depends specifically on the geopolitical boundaries created by counties, it is forced to use an arbitrary and often misleading political jurisdiction as the geographic delimiter of a fluid community structure.

Other approaches have been proposed. In Bridgman's classic publication, *The Rural Hospital,* published by the World Health Organization in 1955 and since reissued, the author proposes that a rural area is "any area such that the time of transport to a built-up area of urban character would exceed one half-hour, and the life of whose population is essentially linked with the working of the soil; the thirty-minute isochrone."[2] This definition underlines two important attributes of rurality. The first is the concept that a rural community is in some way isolated from the resources of urbanity. The changes in the technology of transportation are automatically controlled for by using a transportation standard. Although resources may be available at some distance from the rural community, there are direct and indirect costs associated with moving people and goods. The concept of an isochrone provides a way to identify a coherent geographic area with a relatively homogeneous barrier to the acquisition of urban-based resources. It is of interest that in the guidelines used by the Department of Health, Education, and Welfare (DHEW) to designate health manpower shortage areas to prepare health service plans, the 30-minute isochrone, although not identified as such, is one of the major criteria employed.

The second part of Bridgman's statement refers to the traditional association between rurality and the agricultural profession. This association is no longer as helpful in understanding American rurality; a minority of the American rural population engages in agricultural pursuits, even though the bulk of agriculture still occurs in rural areas.[3] Occupational diversity has come to characterize rural America, and whereas the farmers remain the most tightly organized and politically powerful of the rural constituent groups, they no longer comprise the majority of rural dwellers.[4]

The use of population density to define rurality has the advantage of using a continuous variable that captures more accurately the relativity of the notion of rurality. Tamblyn has used 500 persons per square mile as his cut-off point for rurality; in 1973, approximately 45 million people lived in communities or areas with fewer than 500 people per square mile.[5] The limitations of this method are that it ignores the fact that rural areas are organized into communities with distinctive cultural characteristics, trade patterns, and intercommunity relationships. However, relative population density is certainly a major component of the essence of rurality.

A review of the sociological literature dealing with rural life has difficulty defining the field. In considering hundreds of articles grappling with the various dimensions of rural lives, the reviewers comment that "attempts at definition have ranged from the ecological, to occupational, to attitudinal."[6] Yet no one definition is totally compelling. We feel that it is more logical and more useful to consider the spectrum of rurality, realizing that we must make arbitrary divisions along the continuum in order to handle the concepts in a useful manner. Yet the concept of rurality is an environmental one, the manner in which one lives in relation to nature and its manifestations.

The struggle to define rurality in a statistically satisfying way derives from our need to identify populations with special characteristics and special needs. Such an approach is based on the potentially erroneous assumption that rural areas are systematically different from more densely populated areas and that they therefore share certain basic characteristics. This is a major oversimplification. Rural areas are extremely diverse, with the diversity being a product of regional, cultural, and economic differences. Groups such as native Americans, blacks, and Chicanos are overrepresented in rural locations in the United States. The communities in which these groups live are distinct from a cultural perspective, differing more from one another than they would from a similar cultural group in an urban setting. This cultural diversity must be considered in assessing any rural community, regardless of the density of its population.

In approaching the problem of health status and health care in rural areas, it is important to assess the degree to which rurality as a demographic condition independently influences other population characteristics. A number of studies have been performed that examine the degree to which rurality—however defined—is important in shaping the way people act and think. One of the major issues in the provision of health services is whether or not rural America should be treated as merely an extension of the urban majority, or whether its unique characteristics require a more individualized solution to its special problems. The degree to which rural dwellers differ from their urban counterparts in attitudes and beliefs must be taken into account.

In a recent study performed by Glenn and Hill, an attempt was made to assess the degree to which differences in community population size and population density affect social structure, culture, and personality. The authors report that "survey data from virtually all modern societies reveal remaining rural-urban differences in regard to a variety of kinds of attitudes and behaviors."[3] In their examination of attitudes, they found the community of origin a more powerful explainer of current attitudes than current residence. Thus, urban residents with rural backgrounds retain rural attitudes. The authors support the notion that it is more useful to conceive of a rural-urban continuum, rather than imposing an artificial dichotomous distinction.

This perception is supported by Ford in a comprehensive examination of rural America. The editor notes, "Considerably more remarkable than the mundane (but still valid) observation that people in small rural communities differ from those in the great metropolises is the pattern of gradient differences in social characteristics related to differences in community size."[7] Rural dwellers have a different approach to the solution of problems, and the cadences of their life are different than those of their urban counterparts. Communities and cultures emerge as groups of people confront and solve the unique problems of the places where they live. The rural environment presents a different set of problems than the urban setting, and the solutions that emerge are different. Despite the relative transience and fluidity of American culture, people select and are selected by the environments in which they live. Until very recently the rural population has been the group left behind, a "residual reservoir."[8] As a result, the rural population has tended to encompass many of the disenfranchised members of our country; poor, culturally ignored or estranged, politically naive, often hopeless. As Dillman and Tremblay point out, "The role constraints and more regularized lifestyles enforced by the smallness of the rural community remain, and have been something from which many may feel the need to escape."[9]

Thus, despite the enormous diversity among rural areas, the evidence supports the contention that the beliefs and attitudes of rural dwellers systematically differ from those in more densely populated areas. This view certainly conforms to the popular notion of the craggy, independent farmer, self-sufficient and uncomplaining. Rural dwellers are inherently more conservative, unbending, and independent, living in a social setting where role constraints are more rigid and community interactions more intense and more important.

The persistence of rural singularity in the face of a diverse and heterogeneous culture is supported in an analysis by Fischer of rural opinions as reflected in a wide variety of issues surveyed by national polls.[10] Fischer argues that innovations in social behavior tend to occur in urban settings. The diversity and density of interaction among people at the urban level promotes the interchange of ideas. Urban areas tend to absorb new immigrants. Ideas then diffuse along a population-density gradient into the rural areas. According to this model, rural areas will always retain earlier values, a sort of innate conservatism born of relatively homogeneous populations and diminished opportunity for interaction.

This observation tends to support the growing perception that the "melting pot" ideal of American culture is neither desirable nor factual. Cultural identity is important to people living in a world beset with confusion. Rural people—just like self-contained ethnic groups—are recognizing the value of their way of life and are less apt to apologize for their background. One major justification for the improvement of social services to rural areas is to enable those communities to preserve a valuable way of life. Much of the depletion of rural areas occurred because the mass society implied that rural life was backward and impoverished. Yet the growing unwillingness of people to submerge their distinctiveness in the mass culture has refuted that implicit bias. As Roman points out, "Our nation is not a melting pot, but a bowl of stew."[11]

Given the intuitive perception, supported by observation, that rural dwellers do represent an identifiable group in our society from the standpoint of their attitudes and beliefs, how effective are they in accomplishing their goals through the political process? The traditional rhetoric is contradictory: On one hand, rural residents are seen as having a disproportional influence on the legislative process because they control legislators; and on the other hand, they are seen as powerless and left behind. The first attitude is exemplified by a *New Yorker* article that discusses the ease with which farmers obtain beneficial legislation, as compared with the contortions that New York suffered as it teetered near bankruptcy. "This partiality doubtless reflects the continuing strength of the myth that America is still a nation of people who live on farms or in small towns—or that it should be. . . . Also of influence in federal legislation, of course, is the fact that in the Senate, which can block any bill, the more than eighteen million residents of New York State have the same two votes as Nebraska's population of less than one and a half million. . . ."[12] This contrasts with the conclusion of Knoke and Hering, who studied the political structure of rural America and found that there is "a diminishing political difference between urban and rural.

. . . Leaving aside the possibility of the unforeseen crisis, rural interests are unlikely to capture national political attention."[13]

The situation seems to be best explained by the observation that the agricultural interests are extremely well organized and powerful but that their organizational acumen does not pervade other aspects of rural life. The farm bloc is a relatively homogeneous group, with a long history and a major federal bureaucracy that ministers to it. In other sectors, health included, the inherent internal diversity within rural America, and the dispersed and small size of potential organizational units, frustrates united political action. "Most evidence suggests that there is no rural health system—public or private—distinct from the larger comprehensive health system of our society. This differs considerably from the visible, recognizable rural influence in legislative administrative policy making at all levels of government. Perhaps the so-called farm bloc has a narrowly defined interest in the farm as an economic unit of production."[8]

The importance of the rural ideal is more than convenient political rhetoric. Particularly with the urban malaise of the 1960s and 1970s, there has been deliberate exploration of the notion that population decentralization should be used to combat urban ills.

National policy as reflected in Congressional action demonstrates a commitment to the sustenance of rural America, and repeated attempts have been made to identify rural poverty and underdevelopment and do something about it. The 1970 Agricultural Act underlined the national allegiance to this idea. Title IX of that act stated, "The Congress commits itself to a sound balance between rural and urban America. The Congress considers this balance so essential to the peace, prosperity and welfare of our citizens that the highest priority must be given to the revitalization and development of rural areas."[7] In many ways, this act marked a move away from the categorical concentration on agriculture as the dominant concern in rural America. Congress realized that rural areas lagged significantly in the distribution of wealth, fundamental services, and social amenities. By directing the Department of Agriculture to broaden its mission, it deliberately intervened to improve the social and economic substrate of rural life. Such programs as food stamps and Farmers Home Administration loans to hospitals and clinics are examples of this broader mission.

The lure of rural life is strong. National opinion surveys have shown over the last decade a decided preference among urban dwellers for rural location. Although the dominant American life style is urban, there is a growing desire for the amenities of a rural life style.[14] The studies show that ". . . the desire for a small town or rural setting is extremely pervasive and . . . most respondents view the advantages of living in such a setting even at some distance from a large city as preferable to living in a large city."[15]

There are important reasons why we should be concerned to preserve and improve the quality of rural life. Rural communities are a reservoir of some of those values inherent in our national ethos; they exist as a refuge from the complexity of the cities and as relatively untarnished environmental reserves. Rural living probably also serves as an actual and psychological escape valve for groups and individuals who are overwhelmed by urban life. And of course, certain industries, such as agriculture, that require vast expanses of land will remain primarily rural in location.

Rural is a relative term; dichotomous divisions that separate populations into urban and rural categories may be necessary for comparison, but they ignore the fact that there is a continuum from most rural to most urban. Meaningful definitions of rurality must recognize this gradient.

The salient characteristics of a rural area are its low population density, its distance from urban resources, the relative predominance of an unperturbed natural ecology, and the small sizes of the involved communities. Rural populations in the United States systematically differ from urban populations. Despite rapid social change, transience, and the push toward cultural homogenization, rural dwellers consistently maintain their cultural and behavioral singularity. However, there is marked diversity within rural groups, and some of the most isolated cultural elements in our society live predominantly in rural locations.

The agrarian ideal is a keynote in our political philosophy, and it maintains its primacy in conventional rhetoric. This concept is nourished by a persistent preference on the part of large segments of the urban populations for the rural style of life. Whether this is primarily nostalgic or truly substantive, it has strong normative influence on the maintenance of rurality as a style of life and possible setting in which to live. Rural America continues to play an important part in our economic and cultural life and should continue to be considered an identifiable and worthwhile object of the public concern.

THE RURAL RENAISSANCE—AFTER THE DEMOGRAPHIC WATERSHED

The 1970s marked a dramatic reversal in rural demography. Following persistent decline of rural populations for decades, the seemingly inevitable dissipation of the rural population halted. In language bordering on the exuberant, the Bureau of the Census reported, "For the first time in this century, nonmetropolitan areas grew more rapidly than metropolitan areas (1.2 percent versus 0.8 percent per year) during the 1970s. . . . This development, which began about 1970, represents a reversal of one of the nation's best-established long-term population trends."[16]

The reversal of this deeply imbedded trend toward urbanization is not a reflection of flight from the central city to the suburban fringe. Rather, it is the most remote of the rural counties that are growing most rapidly. As Figure 1.1 demonstrates, the most rural counties, both those adjacent to and those remote from metropolitan areas, are experiencing rapid population growth relative to urban areas. This trend is occurring nationwide; all regions of the country are affected.[17]

As Beale points out, this major new trend does not affect all rural communities. Towns with fewer than 500 people are continuing to lose population through attrition and emigration. The towns with populations between 500 and 2,500 are the ones that are growing most rapidly, with a 16 percent growth rate in the 1960s; and although rural fertility levels remain higher than urban levels—and are greater than the replacement levels—the major rural growth is occurring through immigration.[7]

This remarkable and significant rural demographic renaissance is the result of a number of synergistic factors. As mentioned earlier, there has long been a desire to live in rural areas. But this longing has been largely nostalgic and unobtainable—jobs, cultural stimuli, and social amenities were available only in urban areas. Only recently have a significant number of people been willing or able to act on their locational desires and move into rural areas.

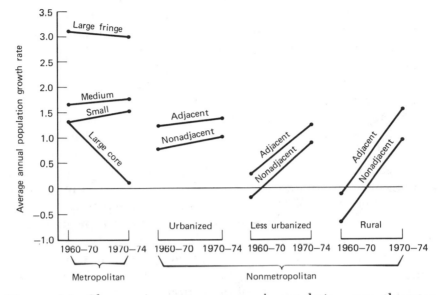

Figure 1.1. Change in average annual population growth rates, 1960–1970 vs. 1970–1974, by county type. (McCarthy RF, Morrison PA: The changing demographic and economic structure of nonmetropolitan areas in the 1970's. The Rand Paper Series, January 1978.)

An additional force that developed the potential for new rural migration is a growing sentiment of anti-urbanism, fueled by a decade of urban unrest and environmental deterioration. A study by Blackwood and Carpenter documents the growing reaction against the anomie and frustration of the large cities and concludes that this anti-urbanism is a definite element in rural migration.[18]

However, these stimuli in and of themselves are not sufficient to explain this rapid and profound reversal of previous trends. A major permissive factor has been the change in the organization of rural life, including major changes in economic structure and cultural proximity to other towns. The completion of the interstate highway system, the improvement in secondary roads, and the growth of scheduled commuter and regional airlines has lessened the isolation of many rural areas.

Perhaps more importantly, decentralization and diffusion of some major economic pursuits to rural areas have taken place. Industrial decentralization has had an impact on rural areas by providing secure employment bases. The energy crisis has forced an increased investment in extraction of previously marginal energy deposits, most of these in rural areas. The growth of rural educational institutions has introduced a significant source of employment into rural areas. In addition to these new economic opportunities has been the growth of a recreational and retirement industry based largely in rural America.[17]

In addition, a perhaps more influential change has occurred in the distribution of services and in rural organization.[19] Complex networks of service industry—perhaps exemplified by the fast-food franchise chains—have diffused into rural areas. The independent, autonomous, and often marginal small-business person in the rural town has been replaced by the hardware store that is part of a nationwide franchising company, with sophisticated inventory control, national marketing strategies, and the availability of management consultation deployed from central offices. Thus, in the economic sphere, rural areas have been much more completely integrated into the economic life of the nation. IBM takes a full-page ad in the *Wall Street Journal* with a picture showing one of its programmers working with the bank's computer in Fossil, Oregon, a town of 540 people. As these economic mycelia penetrate into rural areas, opportunities develop for fairly sophisticated urban dwellers to extend their energies into rural areas. People are able to express their deeply rooted preexistent preferences for rural living.[20]

As might be expected, the new rural immigrant does not resemble those who left for the city. The rural newcomers are not the economic opportunity seekers who went to the city looking for more lucrative jobs, education, or spouses. Rather, they are a better educated, older, and more affluent segment of the population, seeking a better quality of life in a rural area. They are willing to sacrifice a certain amount of earning potential in the transition, as long as they are able to retain a sense of professional challenge and identity in their new location. One-half of these new households have a decreased family income as a result of their move. And, not unsurprisingly, as rural areas once again are attractive magnets for migrants, the spectre of destruction arises; the newcomers may ruin what they have sought by inundation. However, at least for the near future, this new population trend is an invigorating infusion into what many had feared was a stagnant, terminally ill segment of American society.

This marked demographic departure has important implications for the status of rural health care systems. First, it might be expected that the rural pull will extend to some of the health professionals currently in short supply in rural areas. In fact, some of the evidence suggests that this is happening. "New immigrant families tend to be young, small in size, well-educated and concentrated in professional and managerial occupations. . . . Significant numbers of physicians and dentists are among the immigrants in Maine."[21] Although urban locations still attract the majority of newly trained physicians and other health care providers, the appeal of rural living may help deflect part of the stream.

Secondly, diffusion of viable economic operations into rural areas, with sustenance and support from regionalized centers, has promise for health services delivery. Although there are major differences between selling a national brand of fried chicken and providing medical care, some of the organizational lessons from the fast-food franchises are quite applicable to the dissemination and replication of free-standing health care facilities. However, the changing demographic organizational composition of rural society and the increasing attraction of rural life are two major elements that inject substantial optimism into efforts to improve rural health care delivery.

The gradual but seemingly inexorable emigration from rural America reached a watershed in 1970. A demographic rural renaissance is under way, with the most remote areas growing most rapidly. The new immigrants are well educated, seeking improvement in quality of life rather than economic reward. The increasing integration of rural society into the larger economic life of the nation and the proliferation of several new economic endeavors in rural America have permitted these new immigrants to move to rural areas. The same forces that have fueled this renaissance provide a base for improving and transforming rural health care systems.

THE FUNCTION OF HEALTH CARE IN RURAL SOCIETY

Every individual must confront the problems of illness and death. In every society, collective mechanisms evolve to assist the individual in his or her attempts to mitigate the impact of illness. The health care system is the formal expression of society's solution to these challenges. Every society also develops extensive, informal, culturally determined networks that are activated when people define themselves as sick.[22]

In Western culture, we have delegated much of our defense against disease to complex health care systems. In so doing we have developed more effective therapeutic modalities but have become dependent on organizations that are often mysterious and distant— geographically and culturally—from ourselves. Rural communities are particularly vulnerable to the uncertainty this situation can cause because their health care systems are fragile, often controlled by people whose roots and orientations are alien to the community. Yet, paradoxically, it is in rural areas, where greater proportions of the poor and elderly populations live, that health care services are most needed.

Before we begin to explore the state of health and health resources in rural communities, it is important to understand the relationship of health services to the manner in which rural society operates. The function of the health care system is, on one hand, to allow the individual to make use of technological tools available in combatting disease; but perhaps more importantly, on the other hand, it provides a depth of security—real or imagined— that allows people to function in a world full of pain and uncertainty.

Rural societies are characterized by low-density settlement. The sparseness of population is paralleled by a relative paucity of social services. In a country marked by pluralism and abundance, even the wealthiest rural community lacks any back-up to its health care system. The presence of, at best, one system of care in many rural communities makes them vulnerable to sudden, unpredictable interruptions in the provision of this basic social service. This dependence on a fragile service has its effects throughout the social structure. Parsons argues that health and illness are part of the general social equilibrium. "The phenomenon of physical and mental illness and their counteraction are more intimately connected with the equilibrium of the social system than is generally supposed. . . . [The physician] stands at a strategic point in the general balance of forces in the society of which he is a part."[23]

Health care is significantly different from most of the other human services that we use. The medical marketplace has many special characteristics that distinguish it from other social services. Market forces are largely ineffective in distributing health professionals, either in response to population or clinical need. Health services require complex and expensive capital plants, and prolonged training is required for competence in using them. The need for health care is largely unpredictable and often occurs suddenly and catastrophically. Typically, consumers can neither provide for themselves the capability to respond in an emergency nor accurately discriminate among alternative ways of obtaining appropriate assistance.[24]

As a result of this dependence on others for health care, the social organizations that grow up in response to these needs have different characteristics than organizations dealing with education or even fire protection. As the social psychiatrist Fabrega observes, ". . . illness in a fundamental sense reflects an alteration of the body . . . and for this reason also reflects and may trigger an alteration of the fundamental cognitive units that anchor the individual in his world."[25] It is the social disintegration that can be sparked by an inability to deal with illness that makes health care different for most people.

In addition to the importance of health care to individual security, it is becoming increasingly appreciated that health status interacts powerfully with every other important component of rural development. Roemer, a major figure in the field of rural health care not only in this country but internationally, says, "The interdependence of actions in several sectors of health services has become increasingly recognized as necessary for rural improvements. Programs for facility construction, manpower expansion, economic support, and quality promotion are all obviously intertwined. These actions, in turn, are all interdependent with general social changes in agriculture, employment, transportation, education, social security, and other spheres. Reaching goals in any one of these sectors usually depends on parallel actions in several of the others."[26] Investment in rural health systems is thought to have a potential multiplier effect. Healthy rural communities are more likely to have energy to spare for economic development, education, and the other activities that determine community growth.[27]

It is not only in the international arena that this interrelationship has been incorporated into public policy. In the lengthy process of attempting to define the scope and content of the national health planning activities, set in motion by the passage of public law (PL 93–641) in 1976, these issues were specifically considered. In the papers on the National Health Guidelines, it is noted, "Health is seen at the heart of a complex set of interrelationships. Health programs, as it is argued, should form part of a broad program for socio-economic improvements."[28] In a further exploration of the problem of underserved areas in a companion volume, Davis carries the thesis further: "Most medically underserved areas are underserved in other important respects. Human resource development and community development are likely to be deficient as well. If appropriately designed, solutions to the health underservice problem may have important spillover benefits for human resources and community development."[29]

It is widely recognized that provision of health care in rural societies has ramifications beyond the application of technological responses to disease. At a minimum, an adequate health care system is one component of the web of social interactions that makes it possible for people to live and realize their potential in rural areas. However, health care systems may have an even more far-reaching impact, by freeing peoples' energies toward the realization of other broader social goals.

EQUITY: AN ELUSIVE CONCEPT

A rural community requires a functioning health care system for its psychological well-being. Good health is necessary for people to achieve their full potential. Yet the relationship between the health care system and the health of the people it serves is not straightforward, and the amount of health care that should be available to any given community or population group is difficult to determine.

Before turning to a quantitative examination of the state of health and health care in rural America, we must confront the disquieting but plausible notion that health services are tenuously related to health status. More upsetting is the point of view, vigorously presented and defended by Illich, that the health system itself can be a pernicious influence on individual and community well-being.[30] Much of what we discuss later in this book—the means by which we can assure and improve rural health services—is based on the implicit assumption that these health services improve health. It is important to state at the outset that the values underlying the traditional health service delivery system are in flux and that much of what we are attempting to do is provide equity in access to a system that is itself under attack.

The nation, through the health planning law of 1976, committed itself to providing "equal access to quality health care at a reasonable cost."[28] In attempting to flesh out that glowing but imprecise and potentially contradictory goal statement, the authors of the initial discussion papers exhumed the reports of 35 commissions that had been established between 1932 and 1972 to analyze this country's health needs. Their synopsis of those reports is illuminating: ". . . a range of value judgments, personal preferences, political ideology, debatable premises, social and professional perspectives, none of which constitute scientific findings or influences. The word used most often is 'should.' "[28] There is no consensus on what constitutes an adequate, much less an ideal, health system.

A considerable amount of work has been done in an attempt to quantify need, to replace value judgments with valid measures that reflect the interaction between health services and health status. Need, in itself, is not a unitary concept. As Bradshaw points out in his attempt to develop a taxonomy of need, there are at least four ways that governments define need in developing programs.[31] The first level is normative need, that level of service that, in the judgment of experts, is necessary for adequate health services. Although, at the bottom, many of our efforts are guided by our notion of what should be, normative approaches are based on value systems that are difficult to state or defend.

The second level is felt need, more usually expressed as a want. Wants are shapeless and prolific, and like rabbits, they tend to multiply at a distressing rate. Most wants are really normative statements that people make about themselves; our community wants a different level of health care because we are entitled to it. Wants by definition will always outpace resources. In the field of medical care, wants may be a powerful stimulus to political gyrations but often are tangential to more central concerns involved in establishing stable systems.

A third way to approach need is through demand, which is the translation of a want into an effective expressed need. In economic terms, demand is the concerted attempt of a group of consumers to purchase a good or service. Unfortunately, the economics of the health care system is such that it may be very difficult for a rural community to translate a want or need into an effective demand, simply because they are such a small piece of a centralized and capital-intensive marketplace that they lack sufficient economic leverage. In rural areas in particular, people have relatively little control over the money spent by government and other third-party payers on their behalf for health services and thus lack clout in the marketplace.

The fourth level of need is that of comparative need. In this approach, need exists whenever one group has substantially less of something than another group. This technique lends itself to quantification because no matter how much medical care is available, some portion of the population will have less than the average amount. Thus, on October 28, 1978, DHEW could emphatically announce in a press release that "One of every six Americans lives in an area short of primary medical care. . . . Roughly half of the 34 million persons lacking adequate primary care live in cities and half in rural areas. . . . More than 7,000 physicians would be required to serve adequately all designated primary care shortage areas."[32]

By what feat of statistical legerdemain did DHEW define all the areas of need and determine the quantity of resources required to solve the problem? The measure used was the Health Manpower Shortage Area (HMSA), defined as a medical service area with less than one primary health care provider for every 3,500 people. On the face of it, the measure derives from the concept of normative need; an area meeting those conditions has fewer physicians than are necessary to maintain access to health care. But, on closer examination, it becomes evident that in fact a HMSA derives from a comparative measure. By defining the level at one to 3,500, one-sixth of the American people are identified as a target group eligible for federal assistance. Several years earlier the standard had been one physician to 4,000 people; the new standard is partially a response to a gradually increasing supply of physicians that increases the average physician-to-population ratio, and a new concern with physician maldistribution.

In actuality, governmental measures derive from all four types of need. The idea of health manpower shortage areas evolved as a way to define populations eligible for assistance through the National Health Service Corps, a federal program enacted in 1970. The program grew out of the translation of vague community wants into a program designed to allow the federal government to deploy health professionals to communities in need. The Critical Health Manpower Shortage Area (CHMSA), which was the antecedent of today's HMSA, was the tool used to define eligibility. There are literally dozens of similar quasi-statistical measures that are used to focus federal assistance efforts, in agriculature and employment, as well as in health. The very proliferation of such measures in rural health care underlines the futility of attempting to forge agreement on a single unitary definition of need.

It is very important to keep the scope of the problem in perspective. As Somers points out, "The vast, difficult and perplexing problems of the present are seen, in large part, as products of earlier and continuing progress."[33] We have entered into an era where we have the luxury, and suffer the frustration, of dealing with incremental improvements in health care. It is in many ways a by-product of our success that we can split hairs over the optimal distribution of health services, rather than confront the prospect of periodic mass starvation or the devastating pandemics that still afflict much of the world.

Measures of comparative need are partial statistical expressions of equity. Equity in health services is the mainspring that has stimulated the fairly recent broad intervention by federal and state governments into health care. Equity demands both that health services be fairly distributed and that all segments of our population have access to a certain minimum acceptable level of health services, no matter how poor or scattered they might be. Thus equity demands comparability. But it goes further, asserting a collective responsibility ensuring access for all.

Equity is a dynamic concept, changing with time and culture. In an ambitious attempt to measure equity, Anderson and coworkers define equity as that state in which utilization of health services is not affected by social or economic factors.[34,35] Their findings are useful. The major barrier to equitable access to the health care system is the lack of a regular source of care. In the United States, this translates into the lack of a primary care physician who is willing to assume responsibility over time for comprehensive patient care. As Anderson et al. conclude, "By the criteria used here, the group most consistently experiencing inequity in entering the system is the rural farm population."[34] They suggest that a national policy that sought to link all people to a personal provider might be the most efficacious way to ensure equity in health services. This conclusion is very similar to that reached by the National Commission on Community Health Services, which approached the issue normatively. They state, ". . . every patient should have a personal physician who is the central point for integration and continuity of all medical and medically-related services to his patients."[36] Much of the discussion in medical education over the last decade has focused on creating such a physician, a process explored in detail in Chapter 4.

There is no ultimate answer to the question of equity. At the same time we try to determine how to distribute the fruits of our sophisticated medical care system, there is an increasing realization that at least some of those fruits are rotten. Medical care has grown to absorb larger and larger fractions of the nation's wealth, and there does not appear to be a slackening of the trend. Much of the difficulty in obtaining a personal physician can be attributed to the move towards specialization that followed the massive technological explosion in medical care. Iatrogenic disease has become commonplace, and increasing numbers of people are finding themselves estranged from a medical care system that bewilders and impoverishes them. As we move to improve the equitable distribution of medical care in rural areas, we must remember that in some ways rural dwellers are protected from some of the deleterious side effects of a medical care system that has lost touch with the people it purports to serve.

Health is a state of balance within one's environment. Rural people are often more a part of their culture and experience greater control in their daily lives. Part of the challenge of creating rural health care systems is to preserve this independence while improving health services. If we can devise a rural health care system that meshes with the needs, desires, and customs of the community, we may learn to build smaller scale health care systems that can also be effective in urban areas.

REFERENCES

1. *Rural medicine,* proceedings of the conferences held at Cooperstown, New York, October 7 and 8, 1938. Springfield, Charles C Thomas, 1939.
2. Bridgman RF: *The Rural Hospital.* Geneva, World Health Organization, 1955.
3. Glenn ND, Hill L: Rural–urban differences in attitudes and behavior in the United States. *Annals of the American Academy of Political and Social Sciences* 429:36–50, 1977.
4. Brinkman G (ed): *The Development of Rural America.* Lawrence, University Press of Kansas, 1974.
5. Tamblyn LR: *Inequality: A Portrait of Rural America.* Washington, DC, Rural Education Association, 1973.
6. Nolan MF, Hagan RA: Rural sociological research, 1966–1974: Implications for public policy. *Rural Sociology* 40:435–454, 1975.
7. Ford TR (ed): *Rural USA: Persistence and Change.* Ames, Iowa State University Press, 1978.
8. *Rural Health Services: Organization, Delivery and Use.* Ames, Iowa State University Press, 1976.
9. Dillman DA, Tremblay KD: The quality of life in rural America. *Annals of the American Academy of Political and Social Sciences* 429:115–129, 1977.
10. Fischer CS: Urban and rural differences of opinion in contemporary America. *American Journal of Sociology* 94:151–159, 1978.
11. Roman SA: Health policy and the underserved. *Journal of the National Medical Association* 70:31–35, 1978.
12. Around city hall. *New Yorker,* October 1:82, 1978.
13. Knoke D, Hering C: Political structure of rural America. *Annals of the American Academy of Political and Social Sciences* 429:51062, 1977.
14. Hansen, NM: *The Future of Non-Metropolitan America: Studies in the Reversal of Rural and Small Town Population Decline.* Toronto, Lexington Books, 1973.
15. Fuguitt GV: Residential preferences and population distribution. *Demography* 12:491–504, 1975.
16. Population profile of the United States: 1977, in United States Bureau of the Census: *Current Population Reports,* Series P–20, No. 324. Government Printing Office, 1978, p 26.
17. McCarthy RF, Morrison PA: *The Changing Demographic and Economic Structure of Nonmetropolitan Areas in the 1970's.* The Rand Paper Series, January 1978.

18. Blackwood LG, Carpenter EH: The importance of anti-urbanism in determining residential preferences and migration patterns. *Rural Sociology* 43:31–47, 1978.
19. Frisbie WP, Porton DL: The structure of sustenance organization and population change in non-metropolitan America. *Rural Sociology* 41:354–370, 1976.
20. Wardell JM: Equilibrium and change in non-metropolitan growth. *Rural Sociology* 42:157, 1977.
21. Ploch LA: The reversal in migration patterns—Some rural development consequences. *Rural Sociology* 43:293–303, 1978.
22. Kleinman A: International health care planning from an ethnomedical perspective. Critique and recommendations for change. *Medical Anthropology* 2:71–96, Spring 1978.
23. Parsons T: Illness and the role of the physician: A sociological perspective. *American Journal of Orthopsychiatry* 21:452–460, 1951.
24. *Employment Impacts of Health Policy Developments.* Special Report No. 11. Washington, DC, National Commission for Manpower Policy, 1976.
25. Fabrega H: *Disease and Social Behavior: An Interdisciplinary Perspective.* Cambridge, Mass, the MIT Press, 1971.
26. Roemer M: *Rural Health Care.* St. Louis, C. V. Mosby Company, 1976.
27. Golladay FL, Koch-Weser K: The new policies for rural health: Institutional, social, and financial challenges to large-scale implementation. *Proceedings of Royal Society of London. Series B* 199:169–178, 1977.
28. Baselines for setting health goals and standards, in United States Department of Health, Education and Welfare: *Papers on the National Health Guidelines.* DHEW publication No. (HRA) 76–640. Government Printing Office, 1976, p 44.
29. Davis K, Marshall R: Primary health care services for medically underserved populations, in United States Department of Health, Education and Welfare: *Priorities of Section 1501, Papers on the National Health Guidelines.* DHEW publication No. (HRA) 77–641. Government Printing Office, 1977, p 3.
30. Illich I: *Medical Nemesis: The Expropriation of Health.* New York, Random House, 1976.
31. Bradshaw J: A taxonomy of social need, in McLaughlan G (ed): *Problems and Progress in Medical Care: Essay on Current Research.* New York, Oxford University Press, 1972.
32. *HEW News Release,* Health Resources Administration, October 4, 1978.
33. Somers AR: *Health Care in Transition: Directions for the Future.* Chicago, Hospital Research and Educational Trust, 1970.

34. Anderson R, Kravits J, Anderson O: *Equity in Health Services: Empirical Analyses in Social Policy*. Cambridge, Mass, Ballinger, 1975.
35. Anderson R, Aday L: Access to medical care in the United States: Realized and potential. *Medical Care* 16:533–546, 1978.
36. *Health Is a Community Affair—Report of the National Commission on Community Health Services*. Cambridge, Mass, Harvard University Press, 1966.

CHAPTER 2

The Evolution of the Rural Health Care Crisis

The longer we look backward, the further we can look forward.

Dr. Christiaan Barnard[1]

This chapter provides a historical context for understanding the development of rural health care systems from the early colonial period to the present time. Our current system, with its many imperfections and occasional triumphs, is the direct outgrowth of a series of earlier solutions to society's need to minister to the ill and aging. This chapter will lay the groundwork for the presentation of our detailed analysis of the delivery of rural health care in the remaining chapters of the book.

The give-and-take relationship between medicine and social systems has been described by previous researchers and explored in Chapter 1.[2,3] As Sigerist states, "The physician's position in society is never determined by the physician himself, but by the society he is serving."[4] Social and economic developments have at all times had a strong effect on health and disease, and medicine and the other health professions in return have had a considerable impact on society. Each era has had a unique set of medical challenges. Clearly, the rise of American industry in the nineteenth century created a new set of medical problems, both because of the new hazards created by industrialization and the major trend toward urbanization. On the

24

other hand, life in the early American colonies was no paradise; severe epidemics were a predictable part of life with little in the way of medical resources available to modify the ravages of infectious diseases.[5] Roemer has pointed out that the "study of rural medical care is as dynamic as the myriad social and economic forces that shape its character."[6]

The close relationship between medicine and society requires general social improvements (e.g., education, transportation, communication, and employment) as well as changes associated with the direct delivery of health care services to overcome current deficiencies in rural health delivery. Roemer suggests that continued rural health care improvements will depend on future social actions taken by the federal government.[3] Navarro concludes that rural Americans can overcome health care problems by first and foremost gaining control of the resources and wealth they produce.[7] Both are convinced of the strong relationship between health and the social structure. The remainder of this chapter will document this relationship, paying special attention to the current rural health care crisis that, like its predecessors, is the product of the unique social forces of our age. We will review the history of rural health care in the United States during five separate periods:

1. The Colonial Period and the Advent of Industrialization (1620–1850).
2. Industrial Growth and the Pre-Flexner Era (1850–1910).
3. Flexner to World War II (1910–1940).
4. Hill–Burton to the War on Poverty (1940–1970).
5. The Technological Era—the Current Rural Health Care Crisis (1970–present).

THE COLONIAL PERIOD AND THE ADVENT OF INDUSTRIALIZATION (1620–1850)

Colonial America was a rural society. The vast majority of American medicine was provided in rural settings throughout the seventeenth and most of the eighteenth centuries. The first census of the United States in 1790 recorded a population of slightly less than four million.[8] Almost all of this population resided in rural settings; there were only six towns with more than 8,000 residents.

Several accounts have described the health problems of the early colonists.[8,9,10] Those who survived the trip across the Atlantic—in itself a major challenge to health—faced the unknown with respect to the most elemental aspects of life, such as climate and diet.[11] Sites were selected for the earliest colonies not on the basis of public health considerations but for the more pressing reason of providing immediate shelter. Well-trained physicians were in short supply during the early colonial period. Not one physician accompanied the first settlers of Jamestown, and by the first summer in their new home, over half of the settlers had perished.[12]

As one might expect, death and disease were commonplace events for the early colonists. Much of health care delivery in the seventeenth and eighteenth centuries was provided by the women of the household using a distillation of practical experience, home remedies, folk cures, and superstition.[8] Doctors cost time and money and were not called except for serious cases. The self-care movement began in this setting; several self-help medical treatises were very popular in the mid- to late eighteenth century. These books were particularly useful for families that were geographically isolated or financially unable to afford a physician. Two of the most popular books were *Domestic Medicine or the Family Physician: Being an Attempt to Render the Medical Art More Generally Useful with Respect to the Prevention and Cure of Disease,* by William Buchan, and *Every Man His Own Doctor,* by John Tennent.

The earliest physicians in America tended to emulate the prevalent practice of medicine in England rather than initiate new ideas.[10] Medical progress was quite slow, and the physician's armamentarium was scant and of dubious value. Physicians of the 1700s did not understand the basic concepts behind healing, digestion, and cell structure, nor did they have a tradition that allowed them to advance.[13] The practice of purging, cold showers, stimulation of terror, and emetics were actively used by the eighteenth century physician.[12] Many physicians of this period were poorly trained and ill prepared for the responsibility of being the center of the health care "system" in rural areas. The colonial physicians worked as lone tradesmen without the commonplace accoutrements we associate with medical practice—facilities, extensive equipment, and aides. They were itinerant peddlers, purveyors of nostrums and encouragement; but cures were not part of their repertoires.

Prestige in the early colonies was largely conferred on three key individuals—the minister, the lawyer, and the doctor.[14] Although the physician was generally held in lower esteem than either the minister or the lawyer, he was called upon to play an important role in the development of the early communities in America. This leadership role, however, diverted his attention from the practice of medicine, perhaps to the ultimate benefit of his patients.

For most colonial physicians, medicine was more of a trade than a profession.[9] The pay of a physician was uncertain, and a medical practice was often used to supplement another trade such as farming. Three quite different educational paths were available to those seeking a medical career.[15] The most prestigious was the "regular" physician who studied in Europe or Edinburgh and returned to practice medicine and surgery in a major urban center. The prominent physicians of this time, such as John Morgan and Daniel Drake, urged an extensive (4-year) training period for physicians.[12,16] The second and more common path was that of a medical apprenticeship; the aspiring student would live and study with a country physician and his family in a small town for a winter or two.[17] The rapid growth of the country and the demands of the populace did not encourage or require prolonged educations for young men. The quality of the training received by this group of physicians was highly variable, dependent on the skills and interest of the preceptors involved. The third source of medical manpower was the clergy, who played a prominent role in the early New England colonies. Often the clergy, representative of the literate European gentry, were forced into these roles by their fellow townspeople.

Although much attention has centered on the eighteenth-century physicians who obtained European degrees and practiced in the medical institutions in the larger towns, the foundation of colonial medical practice were the country doctors in the small towns and villages.[15] The science of medicine was relatively stagnant during this period, and those discoveries and advances of knowledge in medicine that emerged rarely were incorporated in the practice of the average physician. The country physician was a jack-of-all-trades whose prime attributes were courage and self-confidence. He epitomized the spirit of colonial independence and enjoyed close relationships with his patients. He carried his simple instruments with him on horseback and dispensed medications from his saddlebags.[8] The rural practitioner rarely performed surgery and did so only in emergency situations.[9]

Until the nineteenth century, cities had not grown to the extent where they represented a significant concentration of wealth, and physician maldistribution was nonexistent. In fact, a relative surplus of country doctors fostered considerable competition among medical practitioners, with most physicians being relatively idle except during epidemics.[18] The absence of uniformity in physician training and the rather draconian therapies then in vogue caused many people to turn to quacks for treatment.[15] The medical profession strongly opposed the increasing use of quacks, but had not matured enough as an organized profession to resist the emergence of these new groups of practitioners.

One type of alternative health care practitioner not opposed by the regular physicians was the midwife. Midwives played an important role, particularly among the rural poor, in handling the obstetrical problems facing women of that era.[6,14] Male physicians did not practice obstetrics except in emergencies.[19]

By the time of the American Revolution, there were approximately 3,500 practicing physicians in America, only 400 of whom held formal medical degrees.[12] Until the end of the eighteenth century, university medical training could only be obtained in Europe, but from 1790–1850 a growing number of medical schools and hospitals were established in America. The number of medical schools grew rapidly, from three in 1790 to 35 in 1850; the vast majority were proprietary.[20]

These proprietary schools have been subsequently characterized by medical historians as primarily entrepreneurial ventures of questionable quality. It is clear, however, that colonial society had not matured fast enough to enable the development of a stable, organized medical profession by the early 1800s. The proprietary schools met an important social need—training physicians for the pioneer towns being developed in the West.[21] Mobility had become a national characteristic by the early 1800s, and health care was vital to pioneers in their wilderness experiences. There were not enough physicians to care for the population that was expanding into Kentucky, Tennessee, Ohio, and elsewhere, and the proprietary schools were in part a response to public demand.[8]

During this same period, the number of hospitals in America grew rapidly as well. Before the American Revolution, there were only two hospitals in the colonies; the first was erected in Philadelphia in 1751.[19] This hospital was built and run on the principles of European hospitals, and the primary function of the earliest hospitals in this country was as training facilities for physicians, rather than a way of extending the availability of health care.[22]

Before the early 1800s, hospitals were not intended for private patients. They were for the poor, the homeless, and the mentally ill—a place to be avoided by the gentry.[23] The increase in the number of hospitals over the next 50 years reflected a change in the public's attitude toward hospitals as well as the rapid growth of the population.[24]

With the industrialization and urbanization of America in the mid-nineteenth century, the vast majority of medical enterprise shifted to urban settings. The hospital is an example of the early tendency toward the centralization of medical care. The rural hospital is a recent phenomenon; hospitals built in the first half of the nineteenth century were almost exclusively located in the larger cities and had little impact on the daily routine of the rural physicians of this period.[22]

Two other noteworthy medical developments of the first half of the 1800s were the advent of patent medicines and the spread of the contract system of medical care. Patent medicines were widely advertised in the early 1800s as able to solve the health problems of the common person. The sale of patent medicines flourished in the first half of the nineteenth century as physicians became more professional in their activities and more distant from their patients. Patent medicines were quite capable of easing minor symptoms. Since the major active ingredients were alcohol and a variety of narcotics, they left many medical problems in their wake.[20] Most patent medicines actually were not patented but were very lucrative proprietary ventures on the part of their enthusiastic sponsors.

The contract system of medicine evolved in the early 1800s, especially in the South.[9] Under this system, plantation owners would contract, generally with younger physicians, for the delivery of health care for the workers and residents of the plantation. This system, frowned upon by the older, regular physicians, provided young physicians with a basic income and the experience necessary to advance in the practice of medicine. Ironically, it also provided the slaves of the plantation with better health care than they were to receive after they were freed in the 1860s.

In summary, as the second half of the nineteenth century began, life in America was becoming more structured. The apprenticeship system of medical training was giving way to formal educational preparation, and a growing cadre of physicians attempted—largely ineffectively—to minister to the rapidly growing country.

INDUSTRIAL GROWTH AND THE
PRE-FLEXNER ERA (1850–1910)

After the Civil War, America grew rapidly. Railroads linked the east and west, and large cities began to sprout throughout the nation. The transformation of America from a predominantly rural agricultural nation to an urban industrialized country had profound implications for existing social institutions.[25] Between 1860 and 1900, the proportion of the population that resided in urban areas increased from 19 to 40 percent, bolstered by the influx of immigrants to the larger cities and industrial towns.[10] Major problems that had delayed the maturation of the medical profession before the Civil War—the vast size of the nation, the heterogeneous population spread across a divided country—were no longer seen as barriers.

The medical profession followed the masses of the population to the cities. Wealth had started to accumulate in the larger population centers, encouraging the creation of hospitals, teaching centers, and laboratories. Thus, during the period 1860–1900, urban physicians formed the core of an increasingly organized medical profession.

The medical profession went through a period of transformation during the last two decades of the nineteenth century. The decline in professional morale during the middle of the nineteenth century was replaced by a new-found confidence in medicine.[10] The increased interest in science and research was bolstered by significant financial support from private sources.[11] Much of this energy can be traced to the exciting discoveries of Pasteur and Lister during this period, which for the first time harnessed the scientific method in the service of medical discovery.

Pasteur's work led to the germ theory of disease, which uncovered the role of bacteria and viruses in illness and fostered significant advances in our knowledge of the etiology of communicable diseases. Accurate diagnosis had now replaced sheer guesswork as the key to the practice of medicine.[26] Lister almost singlehandedly "changed surgery from a near massacre to a healing art with the development of antisepsis, absorbable ligatures, and the drainage tube."[11]

What impact did these great discoveries have on the rural general practitioner? The gradual acceptance of the germ theory of disease led to the teaching of localized pathology in medical schools, which in turn led to a dramatic increase in the movement toward specialization. Before 1860, there were no full-time specialists in medical practice. By the end of the century, formal recognition of the medical specialties began to occur, and for the first time the central position of the general practitioner was questioned.[21]

In his classic book, *The Kansas Doctor,* Bonner describes the life and times of the Kansas rural general practitioner during the second half of the nineteenth century.[27] Rural practitioners generally had fewer patients than their urban counterparts, but their day was lengthened by numerous hours on the road visiting patients at home. Bonner discusses the transformation of the country doctor into the town doctor, with the doctor's range of practice gradually decreasing as time went on.

For the general practitioner, surgery was gradually becoming a forbidden art. In the past, most surgery had been simple (e.g., fractures and hernias) and the general practitioner relished the work. With the advances made in surgery due to the experience gained during the Civil War and the work of Lister, the specialties flourished. Stevens concludes that the major problem facing general practitioners at the turn of the twentieth century was their relationship to surgery.[21] One result of this situation was the development of the practice of fee splitting whereby a surgeon would split a fee with a general practitioner who referred a patient.

Hand in hand with the emergence of the medical specialties was the phenomenal growth of the hospital industry in the latter part of the nineteenth century. In 1873, there were approximately 178 hospitals in the United States; in 1909 there were approximately 4,359 hospitals.[21] This surge in the number of hospitals has been attributed to multiple factors—the growth in the population, particularly in the number of wage earners, the development of the nursing profession, the emergence of surgery, and an improved public image of the hospital.[27] The private patient was slowly but surely becoming the primary occupant of the hospital; the hospital was no longer dedicated to caring for the sick poor.[22,28] Specialists were becoming firmly entrenched in the hospitals, and general practitioners, particularly those located in rural areas, were being excluded from this setting.

The increasing loss of patients to city physicians stimulated some individual rural physicians to open hospitals of their own.[29] The small rural hospital, unlike its publicly sponsored urban counterpart, emerged as a private institution primarily for self-pay patients. Typically, it was a proprietary extension of the rural physician's outpatient practice.

The development of the nursing profession during the latter half of the nineteenth century is another good example of the declining status of rural health care. Before the Civil War, most nurses had performed only menial domestic tasks in their jobs. After the Civil War, the progress made in the surgical field along with the rapid growth of hospitals required a more sophisticated level of nursing care.[30]

The ideas of Florence Nightingale dominated the educational and training process for nurses, and a significant number of hospital training schools for nurses were developed. Over 400 hospital nursing schools were started during the last two decades of the nineteenth century.[31] Very few of these, however, were located in small rural hospitals. The hospital with fewer than 100 beds found it quite difficult to give adequate clinical instruction on the wards for student nurses. This eventually caused a shortage of nursing personnel in rural areas as better nurses were attracted to jobs in the larger hospitals in urban settings.

The last two decades of the nineteenth century also saw the emergence of the visiting nurse concept in the cities of the United States.[32] Right after the turn of the twentieth century, Lillian Wald tried to get the Red Cross to take over comparable nursing functions in rural areas.[30] Progress in this endeavor was remarkably slow and reflected the difficulty of effectively channeling resources and personnel to solve rural health problems.

The decline in the relative quality of rural health care was evident at the outset of the twentieth century. Physicians were becoming more and more attracted to the wealthy cities, which contained all the necessary ingredients for a "good" medical practice—a large hospital, the latest equipment, and auxiliary personnel.[18] Formal recognition of the medical specialties began to occur at this time, and the medical profession began to be oriented toward specialties. As Stevens points out, there were major similarities in the problems facing the medical profession in 1900 and 1970, particularly with regard to the role of the general practitioner in a profession increasingly dominated by specialists.[21]

Rural areas were also threatened by the initial federal attempts to standardize hospitals and medical schools in the early 1900s.[24] These attempts have hurt rural areas throughout this century by forcing rural institutions to conform to urban institutional standards.

Despite the deterioration in medical services, life in the country was still considerably healthier than life in the city. The age-standardized death rate in 1900 was 13.9 per 1,000 population in rural areas compared to 20.8 per 1,000 in urban areas.[18] Teddy Roosevelt began his first full term in the White House in 1904 and made attempts to improve rural life through conservation measures as well as his concern for the common person.[11] The first major federal activity dealing with the public's health occurred during his administration with the passage of the Pure Food and Drug Act in 1906.

The early twentieth century marked the first major period of direct federal involvement in the formation of health policy through the passage of health legislation. This contrasted starkly with the lack of federal support for medical care in the nineteenth century and the difficulty the public health movement had in attempting to gain momentum during this earlier period.

FLEXNER TO WORLD WAR II (1910–1940)

At the beginning of the twentieth century, a revolution was initiated in the process of medical education. This revolution was primarily the result of the Flexner report that was published in 1910 at the request and with the support of the Carnegie Foundation for the Advancement of Teaching.[33] Dr. Abraham Flexner spent two years evaluating the medical education system in the United States and concluded

1. There had been a tremendous overproduction of poorly trained physicians.
2. The proliferation of proprietary medical schools was responsible for this overproduction.
3. Medical school expenses had, and would continue to, increase dramatically due to the needs for laboratories.
4. Less expensive medical schools were not justified solely because they allowed access to medical education for the poor.
5. Hospitals under educational control were necessary for medical schools to perform their mission.

Flexner, in essence, wanted to standardize medical education by having fewer, but better run, medical schools producing fewer, but better trained, physicians. The influence of his report resulted in the reduction by half of the number of medical schools in the United States—from 148 in 1910 to 76 in 1932. During the same period, medical education was standardized with the introduction of a three- to four-year curriculum with systematic clinical instruction and increased use of hospital facilities.[5,12] The standardization of the medical education process virtually eliminated rural medical education, as the focus of medical education centered on university departments in large cities.

After World War I, hospitals began to increase in size and assumed their place as the central focus of the health care system. Hospitals had become crucial to the medical education process and, therefore, a critical resource for the aspiring young physician.[22] Physicians, particularly specialists, located near the hospitals, and the inpatient role of the general practitioner was questioned by the medical establishment.

During this period of specialty growth, the first tentative medical group practices were formed. The group practice idea did not take hold rapidly; by 1930 there still were only approximately 150 medical groups in the United States. Most of these groups were in the Midwest and West, and the concept of the group practice of medicine spread slowly as the public and health professionals gained experience with this new mode of practice.

The Great Depression of 1929 hurt all Americans—both rural and urban. The depression had a severe impact on rural general practitioners, most of whom had few paying patients.[2] For those who were able to survive these harsh times, the New Deal of President Franklin Delano Roosevelt brought dramatic changes in the role of the government in public policy and fostered the emergence of the politics of health.

The passage of the Social Security Act in 1935 is a good example of a New Deal enterprise that benefited both urban and rural populations. Among other things, the act provided federal funds for grants to local health departments for programs that provided maternal and child health services as well as crippled children services.[11] For the first time, the federal government took the responsibility of the public's health as a serious concern.

An example of a federal program of this period that attempted to deal with rural health problems was the voluntary prepaid health plan set up by the Farm Security Administration of the Department of Agriculture in the 1930s. The lack of health insurance coverage for those involved with agricultural employment was well known. This program was designed to improve the delivery of medical services to dependent farm families based on a concept of voluntary group action instead of the individual payment of health care bills.[34] At its peak, over 600,000 people in 1,100 rural counties were enrolled in the program, which provided coverage for primary care, surgical, hospital, and dental services.[3]

The program declined by the mid-1940s because too few people joined to make it viable. For the program to have been more successful, it would have had to include all rural farmers as potential members, not just farm families who had been borrowers from the Farm Security Administration.[34] The decline of the program points out the high cost of providing health care to designated segments of rural populations rather than to the population as a whole.

The 1930s was a difficult time for the hospital industry. Despite the increasing power of the medical specialist and the advent of modern medicine with the discovery of sulfa drugs and penicillin, hospitals suffered economically in the period following the depression. Before 1930, the money and initiative for hospital construction depended on localized, private efforts.[3] Largely for this reason, there were very few rural hospital beds. In 1928, 1,200 predominantly rural counties, with almost 15 million people, had no hospital at all.[18]

After the depression, the private construction of health facilities virtually ceased, and over 700 hospitals were shut down during the period from 1930 to 1945.[11] It was not until after World War II that this trend was reversed, with the federal government taking a greater role in the financing and construction of hospitals in the United States.

This period was particularly difficult for rural hospitals. The small rural hospital owned and run by physicians was still common in many rural areas. The ownership of these hospitals was gradually shifted to the community over the next few decades, but their major problems persisted. The small rural hospital had insufficient clinical volume to be able to attract interns or establish a nursing school. Many rural hospitals could not afford to hire nurses, and some had no registered nurses on their staff. Along with staffing problems, concern focused on the outdated equipment in many rural hospitals. Consequently, the quality of care provided at these facilities was questioned. Nonetheless, the small rural hospital remained a critical resource to the general practitioner and the community.

The twentieth century saw the slow growth of organized public health activities in rural areas. In 1912, the first health department in an unincorporated county (Robeson County, South Carolina) was formed; in 1920, 109 of 2,850 rural counties had boards of health.[3,5] Early rural public health activities were quite rudimentary, with a part-time physician usually receiving a small sum of money for occasional services.[35] The Sheppard–Towner Act strengthened rural county health departments in the 1920s by providing federal money for maternal and child health care stations.

The foot soldiers of rural public health were the public health nurses and the sanitarians. The number of public health nurses in America grew dramatically from approximately 200 in 1900 to 3,000 in 1912.[30] By the 1930s, the demand for public health services had grown to the extent that both the federal and state governments intervened in rural public health nursing, reducing the role of voluntary agencies such as the Red Cross.

In general, the scope of rural public health services remained limited during this period. By the early 1930s, only one-fifth of the 2,500 rural counties in the United States had a full-time public health service with fewer than 50 of these having sufficient budget and personnel.[36] The high cost of providing adequate rural public health services was a major barrier. Local rural governments needed outside support to be able to afford an efficient, full-time local health service.[37]

By World War II, rural areas were in a period of decline. The proportion of the overall population living in rural areas was steadily decreasing. The shortage of rural health personnel had become acute. In 1940, only 18.6 percent of health professionals were located in rural areas, a number insufficient to care for the 43.5 percent of the entire population that still lived in rural America.[6] As Flexner had pointed out, a century of overproduction of physicians had not forced doctors into the rural areas where they were needed.[33]

The public image of the general practitioner was also on the wane, eclipsed by the phenomenal growth of the medical specialties. By 1940, over half of all physicians were specialists.[38] This expansion occurred despite the recommendations of such blue-ribbon committees as the National Committee on the Costs of Medical Care that there be four general practitioners for every specialist. The shortage of rural general practitioners caused those remaining physicians willing to live outside the large urban centers to be tremendously overworked.

Rural facilities of this period have been characterized by Mott and Roemer as having "deficiencies in quality, quantity, and above all, by lack of plan."[6] A lack of financial resources and administrative leadership caused most rural areas to be unable to overcome these problems. This situation was not unique to rural hospitals but also existed for other elements of the rural health care system, with a good example being the slow growth of rural public health services before World War II.

In summary, major deficiencies in rural health care were evident in the early 1940s. These deficiencies represented only one part of a far larger problem, the decline of rural America in the twentieth

century. Many feared that rural America would be sacrificed to industrial America.[36]

HILL–BURTON TO THE WAR ON POVERTY
(1940–1970)

The period following World War II was marked by rapid changes
in the medical profession and the hospital industry. With respect
to the medical profession, World War II further accelerated the
process of specialization and centralization. The war had also
forced hospitals to postpone construction and renovation, and attention was focused on the inadequate supply and uneven distribution
of hospital beds, as well as the outdated plant and equipment of many
hospitals. This concern contributed to the passage of the Hospital
Survey and Construction Act (Hill–Burton) in August 1946.

The Hill–Burton program was the largest hospital construction
program ever supported by the federal government. During a 30-
year period, the program provided $4.2 billion in health facility con-
struction subsidies, almost three-quarters of which went to nonprofit
hospitals in the United States.[39] Since no more than 30 percent of
total project costs could be financed by federal subsidies, the Hill–
Burton program stimulated an additional $11 billion investment in
private sector hospital construction. During its period of operation,
the Hill–Burton program was used to finance 30 percent of all hospital projects in the United States and directly accounted for between 10 and 15 percent of the annual cost of hospital construction
in America.[39]

The major goal of the Hill–Burton program was to improve the
supply, distribution, and quality of general hospital beds in the
United States.[40] The original implementation of the program involved a two-stage process. The first stage was a planning stage in
which states assessed hospital needs and developed an allocation
mechanism for distributing funds based on needs. The second stage
involved the dispensing of grants to states for health facility construction including nonprofit general hospitals, specialized hospitals
for the care of patients with tuberculosis and chronic diseases, as well
as public health centers.

The distribution of funds at the state level was made on the basis of the total state population and per capita income. This allocation formula deliberately favored the poorer rural states, particularly those in the South. Within each state, geographic service areas were defined and bed need calculated based on the existing supply of beds and degree of urbanization of the area. The sponsors of the program envisioned that the changes in the hospital system fostered by these policies would lead to an improvement in the supply and distribution of physicians in the country. This latter assumption proved to be incorrect; the program had a marginal impact on physician maldistribution.

With the passage of the most recent health planning law (PL 93–641) in 1975, the Hill–Burton program for all practical purposes ceased to exist. Several retrospective evaluations of the impact of the program have concluded:[39-41]

1. Hill–Burton had a significant effect on the growth in hospital beds per capita.
2. With no controls on the total supply of hospital beds, Hill–Burton may very well have contributed to the excess bed capacity in our current hospital system.
3. Hill–Burton had a major impact on the distribution of state hospital bed supplies.
4. Hill–Burton helped to improve the quality of hospital facilities throughout America and helped to foster the enactment of state hospital licensure programs.
5. Hill–Burton subsidized hospital construction, but its allocative mechanism became increasingly outdated and inappropriate as the program aged.
6. Hill–Burton did *not* significantly affect the distribution of physicians across the country.
7. In the late years of the program, Hill–Burton switched its emphasis from construction to modernization, from rural to poverty areas, and from general hospitals to other types of facilities. These changes were, however, long overdue when they finally occurred.
8. Hill–Burton failed in its attempt to encourage regionalization in the hospital sector.
9. Hill–Burton did not alter the priorities or mechanisms by which American hospitals make decisions.

Increased specialization after World War II accelerated the maldistribution of health professionals and clarified the importance of the concept of regionalization to rural areas. In response to the physician maldistribution problem, a major increase in new medical schools in the period 1950–1970 occurred in rural states such as Kentucky, North Carolina, and Virginia.[42] The maldistribution of physicians also led to a maldistribution of other health professionals, including nurses and pharmacists. The end of World War II coincided with the major shift from private duty to hospital nursing. After 1940, nurses were less willing to work in rural hospitals due to the more attractive employment opportunities available in larger urban institutions.[30]

Early hospital regionalization attempts were made in Maine in the late 1930s and in the Rochester, New York, area in the 1940s, but successful experiments in regionalization have been few and far between.[3] The main problems encountered have been the lack of leadership in rural areas and limited incentives for both urban and rural areas to engage in such activities.

By 1970, three-quarters of all physicians were specialists. This upside-down physician pyramid seemed to augur the eventual extinction of the general practitioner, particularly in rural areas. The Willard and Millis reports of the 1960s and an increasing public inability to gain access to primary care physicians, however, caused a dramatic reversal of this trend.[43] In 1969, the medical specialty of family practice was created as the heir to general practice, and residency training programs were rapidly developed. The year 1970 was significant for the generalist in medicine; it marked the first certifying boards for the new discipline of family medicine.[21]

The organization of medical practice also underwent change in the post-World War II period. The primary location of the physician visit changed from the patient's home to the physician's office or an institutional setting.[44] The concept of group practice finally received the blessing of the American Medical Association in the mid-1960s and slowly spread to medical practices throughout the country. In 1950, fewer than five percent of American physicians were in group practices. By 1969, almost 13 percent of all physicians had adopted this form of medical practice, and the growth has increased since then.[45] The group practice concept developed faster in small towns than in larger cities, because of decreased professional opposition and the greater need to share the overwhelming patient load.[45]

Another significant development of the postwar period was the substantial growth in voluntary health insurance, mainly for the employed and their dependents.[28] In 1943, less than five percent of the United States population had comprehensive health insurance coverage.[6] Improvements in health insurance coverage did not occur evenly across the nation. Large employers were located in the urban centers, and the residents of rural areas either had no health insurance coverage or else had individual commercial policies with higher premiums and fewer benefits than the policies of their urban counterparts.[3] Urban/rural inequities in the health care system were mirrored in health insurance coverage.

Inequities also existed in the programs developed in the 1960s that increased the federal responsibility for the health care of the poor and the elderly. The Medicaid program was initiated in 1965 as an amendment to the Social Security Act of 1935, with a major goal of improving access to health care for the disadvantaged in our country. The program became increasingly unpopular, both at the state and federal level, due to the unexpected astronomical increase in program costs. Davis and Schoen, however, have pointed out that many of the improvements in health care of the poor, such as improved access to care and decreased mortality rates, have been mainly due to the Medicaid program.[46]

The rural poor, however, have not received their fair share of benefits from the Medicaid program. The distribution of Medicaid funds has been extremely uneven. The South has 45 percent of the poor in our country yet receives only 22 percent of the overall Medicaid funds; in 1970 the per capita expenditure for urban children who were Aid to Families with Dependent Children (AFDC) recipients was 15 times greater than for their rural counterparts.[46]

Rural residents are further burdened by the narrow definition of eligibility for most welfare programs as well as the limited range of services available in Medicaid programs in many rural states.[6,42] In general, rural states have been much slower to implement the Medicaid program or to include optional benefits. Despite the significant improvements in health care that can be attributed to the Medicaid program, impoverished residents of rural areas still have substantial access problems in receiving health care, and the mortality rates and incidence of chronic and acute conditions remain disproportionately high among the rural poor.[46]

The Medicare program was implemented in 1965 as an amendment to the Social Security Act of 1935 with the intent of financing health care for the expanding aged portion of the population. During the 1950s and 1960s, the medical profession put more emphasis on the study of chronic conditions with their complex etiologies, and the Medicare program had strong popular support. The program responded to both provider and consumer needs, and despite rapidly increasing costs, it has not been the subject of the same political dissension as that surrounding the Medicaid program until recently.

The program provides almost 40 percent of general hospital income, with an even greater share for the small rural hospital.[3] Nonetheless, rural/urban inequities also exist in the Medicare program. The rural elderly get fewer Medicare benefits yet have a higher incidence of chronic illness than the urban elderly.[46] Evaluation of health care financing programs like Medicaid and Medicare suggest that the key to success is their impact on the organization of medical care at the local level. One would be hard put to conclude that either of these programs has markedly improved the efficiency of the health care system at the local level.[21,46]

To summarize, the problems associated with rural health care continued to mount during the period 1940–1970. These problems have been further intensified in the 1970s due to technological expansion, an uncoordinated set of federal rural health programs, and the fiscal realities of the current times.

THE TECHNOLOGICAL ERA—THE CURRENT RURAL HEALTH CARE CRISIS (1970–PRESENT)

The past few decades have been characterized by major technological advances. In essence, a technological revolution has affected virtually all phases of our lives. A major breakthrough in medical technology occurred after World War II with the practical application of antimicrobial drugs. This dramatic advance has had a major impact on the public's conception of the medical profession and stimulated further changes in medical care.[47]

The use of antibiotics is an excellent example of a *decisive technology* that is cheap, readily available, and results from a thorough understanding of the underlying disease process.[48] Unfortunately, much of the technology that was developed through the heavy support of public funds in the 1960s and 1970s has been referred to by Thomas as "half-way technology."[48] It is makeshift technology that is extraordinarily expensive and often only postpones the inevitable. Examples include heart and kidney transplants and artificial organs.

The fiscal realities of recent years have changed the attitude of the general public toward technological advance. The phenomenal rise in health care costs has been blamed on technology by many critics and has led to cries for slower development of new medical technologies.[49] Whether technology is a major problem underlying rising health care costs is still being debated. Nonetheless, it is clear that technological growth is irreversible and at this point in time not under control.[28] Regulatory efforts, such as the Certificate of Need Program, have not been effective, and the existing cost reimbursement system in fact has stimulated technological advance.[50] Unless major disincentives exist, new technology is rapidly diffused.[49]

How has all this affected rural life? Technological advance has weakened individual control over one's life. It has weakened tradition and the critical values of self-reliance and independence that have been significant parts of rural life in the past.[28,51] It has made many rural people doubt their ability to ensure adequate health care within their own communities.

The modern hospital is an excellent example of the introduction of technology into American society. The role of the hospital has changed during this century from caring for patients to modifying the course of secondary and tertiary medical problems.[47] Significant nonprice competition, in the form of purchasing more and more medical technology, exists in the hospital industry.[52]

With dramatically rising health care costs and the belief that there was an excess of available hospital beds, the Health Resources Administration of the Department of Health and Human Services (DHHS) promulgated the National Guidelines for Health Planning in March 1978. These guidelines stipulate that any given region should have a maximum of four nonfederal, short-term hospital beds per 1,000 population, with an average annual occupancy rate of at least 80 percent. Implementation of the above standards would require a major cutback in hospital bed supply for many local health care systems. This cutback could be accomplished by completely closing or merging inefficient hospital facilities or reducing the number of hospital beds in individual hospitals.

It became clear to the over 50,000 rural constituents who commented on the initial draft of the guidelines that the federal government was going to try to accomplish this overall bed reduction at the expense of small and community hospitals.[53,54] Rural areas would bear the main impact of these regulations despite the major questions still unanswered concerning the true cost savings and efficiency of the plan outlined by the guidelines.

A recent study concluded that savings achieved by the consolidation of hospital facilities according to the DHHS Planning Guidelines would be offset by the indirect costs associated with the management of the program.[55] Furthermore, another study concluded that the misuse of high technology in referral hospitals resulted in $3.7 billion of unnecessary hospital bills in the United States in 1979.[53] This analysis was based on the current trend of increased usage of referral hospitals for treatment of low technology, acute care cases that could easily be treated in small community hospitals.

In summary, the rapid growth of modern technology has led to significant economic growth in our country. In the health care sector, this growth has been accompanied by increased costs and centralization of control and has particularly impaired the ability of rural areas to maintain viable health care systems.[28]

As the supply of rural health services deteriorated in the 1950s and 1960s, the federal government sponsored direct programs to combat further erosion. This activity resulted in the diffusion of federal dollars through a wide variety of programs, and the overall effort has been criticized for duplication and lack of coordination. The list of federal rural health efforts in the 1970s is extensive: National Health Service Corps, Health Underserved Rural Areas Program, Rural Health Initiative, Community Health Centers Program, Appalachian Health Program, Migrant Health Program, a variety of health manpower activities, and, most recently, the Rural Health Services Clinics Act and the Farmers Home Administration rural health facility loan program.

The National Health Service Corps (NHSC) was the first federal effort designed to directly place physicians and other health professionals in rural areas.[56] Since its inception with the passage of PL 91–623 in 1970, the NHSC has increased from an initial budget of $3 million to $140 million in 1979, including a large scholarship program.[57] This financial support has resulted in the development of over 1,000 NHSC sites with more than 2,000 assignees at the present time. As the NHSC has increased in size, it has gone through significant changes in its operation and administration. Its focus has shifted from the development of self-sufficient rural practices to becoming the assured staffing mechanism for other federal rural health projects. The NHSC has become the backbone of the Bureau of Community Health Services (BCHS) strategy for improving rural health care.

By the mid-1970s, the fragmentation of the federal rural health efforts had become obvious, and a strategy was developed for integrating the existing series of categorical programs that affected rural areas.[58] This strategy resulted in the Rural Health Initiative (RHI), and an effort by BCHS to improve health services capacity in rural areas by integration of the resources that it controlled. In reality, resource integration meant that a single site could receive funds from several federal programs at the same time in its effort to develop primary care capacity at the local level. The key to the RHI strategy was the appropriate coordination of resources (e.g., manpower, equipment, and facilities) available through the NHSC and the Community Health Centers programs. The Community Health Centers program was an outgrowth of the poverty programs of the 1960s and supported primary care projects in both urban and rural settings in the 1970s.

The RHI grew in size from $7.2 million in 1975 to $63.7 million in 1980. However, the program lacks a statutory base and has come under increasing criticism in recent years, particularly from the supporters of the individual categorical programs. In addition, the reduced attention paid to the economic self-sufficiency of RHI sites has soured Congress on this type of approach since legislators are afraid they will be asked to fund the same projects in perpetuity.

A parallel and somewhat complementary effort to the RHI was the Health Underserved Rural Areas Program (HURA). HURA was a project grant program for rural health research and demonstration and allowed for experimentation with alternative health services delivery models for underserved populations in rural areas.[59] Although its budget increased from $3.3 million in fiscal year 1975 to $16.5 million in fiscal year 1979, HURA has not produced the innovative results that were expected from this demonstration and evaluation program and has been recently reorganized into the Primary Care Research and Demonstration (PCRD) grant program. PCRD is intended to support research and demonstration projects that can improve operational aspects of the RHI, although the future of the program is in doubt.

The past decade has witnessed a variety of federal rural programs targeted at specific populations. Among these efforts to develop local health care capacity have been the Migrant Health Program and the Appalachian Health Program. There are currently over 100 Migrant Health Clinics and 200 grantees of the Appalachian Health Program whose efforts are sometimes coordinated with the Rural Health Initiative.

The 1970s saw the enactment of extensive federal legislation emphasizing the training of physician and nonphysician personnel for the delivery of primary care. In the early 1970s, the emphasis of federal legislation was on providing fiscal stability to health professional schools through construction grants, capitation support, and a variety of special project grants, most notably those emphasizing the role of the primary care practitioner.

In 1976, with the passage of PL 94–484 (Health Professions Educational Assistance Act), the federal government attempted to exercise greater control over the training of physicians by tying the receipt of capitation and other federal training support to the distribution of residency positions in medical schools.[60] With geographic and specialty maldistribution having replaced the shortage of physicians as the major health manpower policy issue, the federal government wanted to ensure that at least half of the available first-year residency slots for physicians would be in primary care specialties. Extensive funds were also directed to special project grants for primary care training and service delivery programs. These efforts greatly accelerated the emergence of family medicine, resulting in the development of family practice programs in almost 90 percent of United States medical schools and a dramatic increase in the number of family practice residents from 290 in 1970 to 5,421 in 1977.[61] In addition, over 20,000 graduates of federally funded nurse practitioncr and physician assistant programs have completed their training with slightly less than three-quarters practicing primary care.[62]

This reemphasis of the generalist role in the health care system has led to improvements for rural health care delivery. Well over half of the graduates of family practice residencies practice in towns with less than 25,000 population; nonphysician personnel, particularly physicians' assistants, locate proportionately more in rural areas than their physician counterparts.[61,62] Despite these gains, and a rapidly growing surplus of physicians and other health professionals, there has not been significant improvement in the geographic distribution of health personnel.[63,64] The number of practitioners in each of the major health professions is predicted to increase from 40 to 70 percent from 1975 to 1990, yet progress in the recruitment and retention of health personnel for rural areas is still quite slow.[63]

One final piece of federal legislation that points out the difficulty of implementing changes in rural health care systems is the Rural Health Services Clinic Act (PL 95–210) of 1977. This act amends Titles 18 and 19 of the Social Security Act to permit Medicare and Medicaid reimbursement to rural clinics staffed by physicians' assistants and nurse practitioners.

Despite high hopes, implementation of the law has proceeded at a very slow pace, with only a small proportion of clinics participating, many states unwilling to promote the program, and several clinics even withdrawing from the program after having been certified. The main reasons for the lack of success of this program have been inertia, strained state Medicaid budgets, complexities of the cost reimbursement formula, excessive paperwork, inadequate patient load to make certification worthwhile, and opposition by physicians.[65] Despite passage of a good law with sound intentions, little impact has been achieved due to difficulties with the practical implementation of the law.

Finally, it is also worth noting a few of the myriad other attempts that have been made in the past decade to improve rural health care capabilities. Among these are

1. Federal programs, such as those spawned by the HMO Act of 1973 and the National Health Planning and Resource Development Act (PL 93–641) of 1975. The HMO Act has had minimal

impact on rural areas despite its priority for development of health maintenance organizations in rural areas. The Planning Act, although at first accepted in theory, has not been practically applied and, if anything, has hindered progress in rural areas as indicated by our earlier discussion of the misapplication of the National Health Planning Guidelines.

2. State programs that have promoted specific types of rural health care activities, the most prominent being activities related to the recruitment and retention of primary care practitioners.[66] These programs have been developed in an increasing number of states with varying degrees of success. A very successful state program has been the one developed in North Carolina under the auspices of the Office of Rural Health Services.

3. Foundation efforts to develop innovative rural health care systems in underserved areas. Paramount among these efforts are the development of physician/administrator teams at clinics sponsored by the Rural Practice Project of the Robert Wood Johnson Foundation and the Innovations in Ambulatory Primary Care program supported by the W. K. Kellogg Foundation.[67,68]

4. Private groups that have contracted with individual communities to provide health manpower and services to rural areas for a fixed sum of money. An example of this type of private venture is Health Systems Research Institute, a Utah based firm.[56] As can be expected, these types of private arrangements are expensive and best suited for wealthy rural communities.

In summary, there is currently a rural health care crisis in our country. Rapid technological advances in all phases of life, including medicine, have undermined certain aspects of rural life. There remains a large gap between the growth of modern technology and its social application, particularly in rural areas.[6] Many rural programs have been developed without sufficient thought given to the rapid changes occurring in technology and their consequences for rural dwellers.[51] Programs developed at the federal, state, and other levels to address rural health care needs generally have dealt with immediate, pressing concerns rather than coming to grips with the true, underlying problems of rural health care.[51] As Davis and Marshall have indicated, "placing physicians in a shortage area and charging prevailing rates for services may have little impact if the major deterrents to appropriate utilization of primary health services are poverty, lack of transportation, and fear or distrust of health professionals alien to the culture of the area."[69]

Solutions to the rural health crisis will not be simple. Health care delivery reform and other rural development improvements are inexorably intertwined. Rural life is characterized by lack of employment opportunity; inadequate housing, education, transportation, and limited waste management systems; fragmented planning and lack of local leadership; insufficient capital investment and credit availability; and limited public revenue available to local governments.[51,70] When these problems are combined with the weak lobbying efforts on behalf of rural development, the minimum population levels often necessary to support efficient social service programs, and the energy crisis, the issue becomes even more complex.[51,71,72]

Viewed within the context of American history, the rural health care dilemma is nothing new. Ever since the urbanization process siphoned off human resources from rural communities, rural areas have tended to lag behind in their efforts to provide up-to-date health services. Certain historical trends that emerge from our review are worth noting as we contemplate future efforts to improve rural health care services.

First, the relative supply of physicians appears to be cyclic. We have gone from periods of physician shortage to surplus and back again. The colonial period started with shortage and ended with too many physicians trained in the apprentice mode. The shortage of the industrial period was erased by the production of proprietary medical schools and then reappeared once the Flexnerian reforms were fully implemented. We are once again on the verge of surplus as the result of direct governmental attempts to increase the aggregate supply of physicians. It is not clear how long the current phase will last.

Societal forces, the organization of human services, and the centralization of wealth appear to be more significant factors than the total number of health professionals in distributing doctors. Physicians with the skills and orientation of the generalist are more inclined to settle in smaller towns. Only by maintaining a reasonable balance between generalists and specialists can we assure that there will be a manpower pool from which rural communities can draw.

Government intervention is effective in accelerating the process of social change. However, it is not apparent that legislative programs alone initiate change. The study of rural health care shows that government has tended to go from crisis to crisis, responding after the fact to wide-spread social perceptions that something is awry. Government programs, once initiated, tend to be rather ponderous and inflexible but can have significant effects in changing the rural health care system.

As this book is being written, we seem to be entering an era marked by disenchantment with government intervention. Many of the rural health programs of the 1970s are slated to be dismantled. In a totally unregulated environment, rural areas will fare poorly in the technological wars. The only reassurance we can draw from history is that this reaction will generate its own response and we will witness another cycle and another set of solutions.

REFERENCES

1. Johnston W: *Before the Age of Miracles.* New York, Paul E. Erickson Inc., 1972.
2. Rosen G: *From Medical Police to Social Medicine—Essays on the History of Health Care.* New York, Science History Publications, 1974.
3. Roemer M: *Rural Health Care.* St. Louis, C. V. Mosby Company, 1976.
4. Marti-Ibanez F (ed): *Henry E. Sigerist on the History of Medicine.* New York, MD Publications, 1960.
5. Sigerist H: *American Medicine.* New York, W. W. Norton and Company, 1934.
6. Mott F, Roemer M: *Rural Health and Medical Care.* New York, McGraw-Hill, 1948.
7. Navarro V: Political and economic determinants of health and health care in rural America. *Inquiry* 13:111–121, 1976.
8. Pickard M, Buley R: *The Midwest Pioneer—His Ills, Cures, and Doctors.* New York, Henry Schuman, 1946.
9. Duffy J: *The Healers.* New York, McGraw-Hill, 1976.
10. Shryock R: *Medicine in America—Historical Essays.* Baltimore, Johns Hopkins University Press, 1966.
11. Hill L: Health in America—A personal perspective, in: *Health in America: 1776–1976.* U.S. Government Printing Office, 1976.

12. Dolan J, Adams-Smith W: *Health and Society*. New York, Seabury Press, 1978.
13. Flexner J: *Doctors on Horseback*. New York, Viking Press, 1937.
14. Packard F: *History of Medicine in the United States*. New York, Hafner Publishing Company, 1963.
15. Bell W: *The Colonial Physician and Other Essays*. New York, Science History Publications, 1977 (second printing revised).
16. Bell W: *John Morgan—Continental Doctor*. Philadelphia, University of Pennsylvania Press, 1965.
17. Drake D. *Practical Essays on Medical Education and the Medical Profession in the United States*. Baltimore, Johns Hopkins University Press, 1952.
18. Roemer M: Historic development of the current crisis of rural medicine in the United States, in Kagan S (ed): *Victor Robinson Memorial Volume*. New York, Froben Press, 1948.
19. Beck J: *Medicine in the American Colonies*. Albuquerque, Horn and Wallace, 1966.
20. Risse G, Numbers R, Leavitt J (eds): *Medicine Without Doctors*. New York, Science History Publications, 1977.
21. Stevens R: *American Medicine and the Public Interest*. New Haven, Conn, Yale University Press, 1971.
22. Rosenberg C: The origins of the American hospital system. *Bulletin of the New York Academy of Medicine* 55:10–21, 1979.
23. Marks G, Beatty W: *The Story of Medicine in America*. New York, Charles Scribner & Sons, 1973.
24. Shryock R: *The Development of Modern Medicine*. Philadelphia, University of Pennsylvania Press, 1936.
25. Rosen G: *Preventive Medicine in the United States: 1900–1975*. New York, Prodist, 1977.
26. Thomas L: *The Medusa and the Snail*. New York, Viking Press, 1979.
27. Bonner T: *The Kansas Doctor*. Lawrence, University of Kansas Press, 1959.
28. Somers A, Somers H: *Health and Health Care: Policies in Perspective*. Germantown, Aspen, 1977.
29. Hertzler A: *The Horse and Buggy Doctor*. New York, Harper and Bros., 1938.
30. Bullough V, Bullough B: *The Care of the Sick: The Emergence of Modern Nursing*. New York, Prodist, 1978.
31. Shryock R: *The History of Nursing*. Philadelphia, W. B. Saunders Company, 1959.
32. Winslow C: *The Evolution and Significance of the Modern Public Health Campaign*. New Haven, Conn, Yale University Press, 1923.

33. Flexner A: *Medical Education in the United States and Canada.* New York, The Carnegie Foundation for the Advancement of Teaching, 1910.
34. Goldman F: Medical care for farmers. *Medical Care* 3:19–35, 1943.
35. Freeman A (ed): *A Study of Rural Public Health Service.* New York, Oxford University Press, 1933.
36. Winslow C: *Health on the Farm and in the Village.* New York, MacMillan Company, 1931.
37. Lumsden L: Extent of rural health service in the United States: 1926–1930. Public Health Reports 45:1065–1081, 1930.
38. Rosen G: *The Specialization of Medicine with Particular Reference to Ophthalmology.* New York, Froben Press, 1944.
39. Feshbach D: What's inside the black box: A case study of allocative politics in the Hill–Burton program. *International Journal of Health Service* 9:313–339, 1979.
40. Clark L, Field M, Koontz T, Koontz V: The impact of Hill–Burton: An analysis of hospital bed and physician distribution in the United States. 1950–1970. *Medical Care* 18:532–550, 1980.
41. Lave J, Lave L: *The Hospital Construction Act: An Evaluation of the Hill–Burton Program, 1948–1973.* Washington DC, American Enterprise Institute for Public Policy Research, 1974.
42. Roemer M, Anzel D: Health needs and services of the rural poor. *Medical Care Review* 25:371–390, 461–491, 1968.
43. *The Report of the Citizens Commission on Graduate Medical Education, The Graduate Education of Physicians*, Chicago, American Medical Association, 1966.
44. Rosenberg C: The therapeutic revolution: Medicine, meaning, and social change in nineteenth century America. *Perspectives in Biology and Medicine* 20:485–506, 1977.
45. Roemer M, Mera J, Shonick W: The ecology of group medical practice in the United States. *Medical Care* 12:627–637, 1974.
46. Davis K, Schoen C: *Health and the War on Poverty: A Ten Year Appraisal.* Washington DC, Brookings Institution, 1978.
47. Saward E: The current role of the hospital in ambulatory care. *Bulletin of the New York Academy of Medicine* 55:112–118, 1979.
48. Thomas L: *The Lives of a Cell.* New York, Viking Press, 1974.
49. Altman S, Blendon R (eds): *Medical Technology: The Culprit Behind Health Care Costs?* USDHEW, Public Health Service, 1979.
50. Russell L: *Technology in Hospitals: Medical Advances and Their Diffusion.* Washington DC, Brookings Institution, 1979.
51. *The People Left Behind—A Report by the President's National Advisory Committee on Rural Poverty.* Washington DC, 1967.

52. *NCHSR Research Proceedings Series*. Medical Technology. USDHEW, NCHSR, September 1979.
53. Crozier D (ed): *The Human-Size Hospital* 2:1–4, 1980.
54. Danaceau P: *The Health Planning Guidelines Controversy: A Report from Iowa and Texas*. USDHEW, Health Resources Administration, 1979.
55. Schwartz W, Joskow P: Duplicated hospital facilities—How much can we save by consolidating them. *New England Journal of Medicine* 303:1449–1457, 1980.
56. Kane R, Dean M, Solomon M: An evaluation of rural health care research. *Evaluation Quarterly* 3:139–189, 1979.
57. Rosenblatt R, Moscovice I: The National Health Service Corps: Rapid growth and uncertain future. *Milbank Memorial Fund Quarterly* 59:283–309, 1980.
58. Rockoff M, Gorin L, Kleinman J: Positive programming: The use of data in planning for the rural health initiative. *Journal of Community Health* 4:204–216, 1979.
59. Samuels M: Federal strategy for rural health: A systems approach. *Annals of New York Academy of Science* 310:163–168, 1978.
60. LeRoy L, Lee P: *Deliberations and Compromise: The Health Professions Educational Assistance Act of 1976*. Cambridge, Mass, Ballinger, 1977.
61. Geyman J: Family practice in evolution: Progress, problems and projections. *New England Journal of Medicine* 298:593–601, 1978.
62. Congressional Budget Office: *Physician Extenders: Their Current and Future Role in Medical Care Delivery*. U.S. Government Printing Office, April 1979.
63. *A Report to the President and Congress on the Status of Health Professions Personnel*. USDHEW, Bureau of Health Manpower, August 1978.
64. *Report of the Graduate Medical Education National Advisory Committee to the Secretary, DHHS*. U.S. Government Printing Office, September 1980.
65. *Health Law Newsletter*. National Health Law Program, Issue No. 90:2–3, 1978.
66. Sheps C, Bachar M: Rural areas and personal health services: Current strategies. *American Journal of Public Health* 71 (suppl):71–82, 1981.
67. Madison D: *Starting Out in Rural Practice*. Department of Social and Administrative Medicine, University of North Carolina at Chapel Hill, 1980.
68. *1977 Annual Report*. W. K. Kellogg Foundation, Battle Creek, Michigan, 1977.
69. Davis K, Marshall R: Primary health care services for medically underserved populations, in: *Papers on the National Health Guidelines—The Priorities of Section 1502*. U.S. Government Printing Office, 1977.

70. Policy statements offered for APHA. *The Nation's Health*, September 1977.
71. Davis K, Marshall R: New developments in the market for rural health care, in Scheffler R (ed): *Research in Health Economics, Volume 1*. Greenwich, Conn, JAI Press, 1979.
72. Myers B: Health care for the poor, in Levin A (ed): *Health Services: The Local Perspective*. Proceedings of the Academy of Political Science, New York, 1977.

CHAPTER 3

Health Status and Health Resources in Rural America

Health care is crucial to the maintenance of a functional rural community. Because sparseness of population and the relative lack of human resources are central characteristics of rural life, rural health care systems are more fragile than their urban counterparts. This chapter explores the degree to which rural inhabitants actually experience different levels of health status than the rest of the population and examines the disparity in available health care resources between rural areas and the larger society.

The methodological problems of measuring health status are in themselves immense. A vast literature deals with the difficulty of describing health status in a useful, valid, and reliable way, and there is an abundance of instruments proposed for doing so in a quantitative manner.[1] Part of the problem stems from an inability to measure health. Health is a subjective state, the organism's experience of being in a state of homeostatic balance internally and with its environment. Yet health is usually measured in terms of the absence of disease, and the relative health status of a community is expressed in terms of the prevalence within a population of certain measures of sickness or death.

The exact relationship between medical care and health status is elusive.[2] The major determinants of health are intrinsic and environmental, the interaction between the individual's genetic potential and the sustenance and insults residing in the immediate environment. Health care, particularly those health services delivered by physicians and hospitals, is directed for the most part at preexisting symptoms. For all the recent emphasis on holistic medicine and prevention, the health care system exists to deal with complaints. People go to doctors when they feel sick. Since the majority of illnesses are self-limited and resolve spontaneously without intervention, identifying the actual contribution of health services is obscured by the fact that relatively inconsequential conditions form the majority of medical practice.

The major measures of health status are insensitive to minor fluctuations in the state of a population's well-being. Mortality statistics, although they have the advantage of cataloguing an easily observed and usually unambiguous event, change only slowly as the result of an improvement in health status. Other measures, such as infant mortality, are used as surrogates for the health status of entire populations, although they focus on only one age spectrum within the population. Infant mortality rates are more sensitive to changes in health status and health resources than gross mortality rates but remain indirect measures of health status.

Even given the relative crudity of these measures, there have been major improvements in the United States in measures of health status. Mortality rates have fallen; life span has increased. Yet it is impossible to attribute these changes to any specific intervention. So many forces are at play in determining life span or infant mortality—ranging from the state of the water supply to the amount of saturated fats in diets to changes in the speed limit—that the exact contribution of health services per se to health status cannot be isolated. As we review the available statistical data comparing the health status and health resources of rural areas with more urbanized areas, we must be cautious in our attempts to attribute the perceived variations to any narrow set of possible causes.

RURAL HEALTH STATUS

Table 3.1 examines infant and maternal mortality rates for metropolitan and nonmetropolitan areas and illustrates changes in the

TABLE 3.1. Infant Mortality Rates and Maternal Mortality Rates by Residence

	Metropolitan Area			Nonmetropolitan Area		
Category	1968	1969–73	1974–77	1968	1969–73	1974–77
Deaths Per 1,000 Live Births						
Infant mortality rates	21.1	18.8	15.2	23.0	20.7	16.2
White	18.6		13.3	20.2		14.5
Non-white	32.5		24.9	39.3		27.6
Deaths Per 100,000 Live Births						
Maternal mortality rates	23.6			26.4		

Source: Adapted from Mathews, *Health Services in Rural America*, U.S. Department of Agriculture, Rural Development Service and Economic Research Service, Agriculture Information Bulletin No. 362, April 1974, page 17, Table 14, Ahearn, *Health Care in Rural America*, U.S. Department of Agriculture, Economics, Statistics, and Cooperatives Service, Agriculture Information Bulletin No. 428, July 1979, page 23, Table 10; and *Health, United States, 1980*, DHHS Pub. No. (PHS) 81–1232, December 1980, page 31, Table A.

infant mortality rate over the last decade. Infant mortality rates have been falling steadily in the United States, most likely as a result of improvement in the general sociodemographic status and in the care of low-birth-weight infants, the major group at risk for infant death. Despite this falling rate, rural areas demonstrate a higher infant mortality rate for all three time periods studied and continue to lag behind metropolitan areas. Maternal mortality, a rarer but much more devastating event, is also higher for rural areas. It is notable that race has a more powerful association with mortality rates than residential location, bolstering the conclusion that economic, sociological, and biological factors are of prime importance in determining health status. White rural residents, for example, have a much lower infant mortality rate than do black urban residents. Yet rural residents experience higher infant mortality rates even after correcting for race, a finding that may very well be attributable to less adequate health care services in rural areas.

In many ways, health status is better measured by assessing the functional status of individuals, either as reflected in their own appraisal of their current condition or by measuring the number of days in which they are restricted from performing their usual activities. Tables 3.2 through 3.4 provide some insight into the relative functional capability of rural dwellers and tend to corroborate the conclusions that are suggested by the disparities in the infant mortality rates. Table 3.2 sugggests that rural dwellers consistently have an equal or higher prevalence of serious chronic health conditions in comparison to urban persons. The material presented in the second part of the data, however, runs counter to what one might expect. For a series of common acute causes of illness, rural dwellers experience a lower rate of disability as measured by days spent in bed. These data may reflect not health status, but the propensity of rural dwellers to continue to work despite acute intercurrent illnesses or injuries.

Table 3.3 tends to reinforce the latter interpretation. In this table, days of restricted activity are adjusted for age and then displayed for the major regions of the country and the rural and urban areas within them. The table demonstrates that there are significant regional impacts on disability and that location of residence has a powerful but not totally consistent effect. The rural South stands out as the rural area of the country with highest reported rates of re-

TABLE 3.2. Comparison of Rural and Urban Health Statistics for Selected Health Conditions

Chronic Conditions	Prevalence per 1,000 Persons	
	Urban	Rural
Hypertension	58.7	62.6
Chronic bronchitis	33.0	33.0
Coronary heart disease	16.2	16.6
Ulcer of stomach and duodenum	15.9	18.9
Hernia	15.3	17.6
Hypertensive heart disease	9.6	12.0
Gallbladder disease	9.0	12.5
Emphysema	5.4	8.8

Acute Conditions	Days of Bed Disability per 100 Persons per Year	
	Urban	Rural
All acute conditions	415.2	376.3
Respiratory conditions	317.5	259.0
Influenza	110.8	102.4
Injuries	66.1	65.8
Infective diseases	47.3	38.1
Digestive system conditions	21.3	19.5

Source: Adapted from Kane, *Problems in Rural Health Care* in *Health Services: The Local Perspective.* Praeger, New York, 1977, page 137, Table 2.

TABLE 3.3. Age-Adjusted Days of Restricted Activity per Person per Year, by Geographic Region: United States, 1973, 1974

	All Areas	SMSA[a]		Non-SMSA
		Central City	Noncentral City	
All regions	16.8	18.3	15.7	16.7
Northeast	14.3	16.6	12.9	13.6
North Central	15.9	17.2	15.4	15.2
South	18.8	19.1	17.1	19.4
West	18.6	21.1	18.4	15.0

Source: U.S. Department of Health, Education, and Welfare, National Center for Health Statistics, unpublished tabulations.

[a]SMSA: Standard Metropolitan Statistical Area.

stricted activity days. The only entirely consistent finding is that in every region of the country, rural and central city dwellers have higher rates of restricted activity than their counterparts within the more affluent portions of the urban landscape.

Table 3.4 presents the self-evaluation of health status by elderly rural and urban dwellers and also demonstrates the interrelationship between economic status and disability. It is clear that elderly people who receive federal old age assistance through the Social Security Administration experience a much lower level of good health than their elderly counterparts who do not receive assistance. Once again, there is a rural–urban gradient, with rural dwellers rating themselves as being in poorer overall health even after taking their economic conditions into consideration. However, as in the case of race, socioeconomic status appears to have a greater overall impact than residence alone, although the rural effect persists even after correction for race and socioeconomic status.[3]

Putting these diverse sets of data together does not yield an unambiguous answer to the question of whether it is less healthy to live in a rural area. Other studies have demonstrated that the rural nonfarm population has a higher injury rate than others and that rural blue collar workers experience greater occupationally related injuries and work lost.[4] Rural areas are a reservoir of the poor and the elderly, and these groups have relatively impaired health status. It is impossible to conclude that living in rural areas per se is unhealthy, and some evidence seems to point in the opposite direction. However, because of the demographic composition of rural areas—greater numbers of the old, the black, and the poor—it is reasonable to conclude that the need for health services is greater in rural America.[5]

RURAL HEALTH RESOURCES

The relative deficiency of health care resources in rural areas is unambiguous. Despite evidence that the need for health care services is greater for rural populations, our current health care system is unable to translate that need into effective demand. In a nationwide attempt to determine residual inequities in the health care sys-

TABLE 3.4. Self-Evaluation of Health Status by Elderly Rural and Urban Dwellers, 1973

Respondents with Characteristic	Recipients of Old Age Assistance				Nonrecipients			
	Farm or Open Country	Small Town	Small City	Large City	Farm or Open Country	Small Town	Small City	Large City
Total number (in thousands)	378	554	225	475	2,561	4,478	2,422	4,136
Self-rating of health as poor (%)	59.9	51.3	43.4	43.1	29.0	20.4	19.0	21.2
Five or more health disorders (%)	50.7	49.9	43.0	40.2	30.1	24.9	34.3	22.3
Severe physical activity limitation (%)	46.4	50.0	48.1	41.5	29.7	22.7	25.3	21.0
Mean number of health disorders (%)	5.27	5.20	4.81	4.59	3.94	3.55	3.58	3.27

Source: Adapted from Social Security Bulletin, June 1978, Vol. 41, No. 6, page 20, Table 4; HEW Publication No. (SSA) 78–11700.

tem, Andersen and his coauthors conclude, "By the criteria used here, the group most consistently experiencing inequity in entering the system is the rural farm population. They are less likely than the rest of the population to be admitted to a hospital or to see a doctor or a dentist. Access problems for inner city residents appear in contrast less serious."[6] Thus, despite the fact that inner-city residents seem to share some of the same health status disadvantages as rural inhabitants, they do have more ready access to health facilities.

Tables 3.5 through 3.7 and Figure 3.1 exhibit the relative supply of health professionals in the United States, with particular attention to regional and residential disparities. The health care system in the United States is pyramidal, with physicians forming the base of the pyramid. Private medical practice is the norm in the country, and most people gain access to the medical care system by consulting private physicians. Physicians act as brokers on behalf of their patients, selecting from a growing array of diagnostic and therapeutic interventions that they control. Laboratory examinations, hospital care, a variety of nursing services, physical therapy, and rehabilitative services are deployed in response to physician orders. The physician acts as the gatekeeper to the medical care system.

Table 3.5 illustrates the maldistribution of physicians within the United States. Although regional differences exist, they are relatively minor when compared to the dramatic tendency of physicians to cluster in metropolitan areas. There are fewer than half as many physicians serving equivalent populations in rural as opposed to urban areas. And although the aggregate supply of physicians in relation to population is expanding rapidly—Table 3.5 demonstrates a 10 percent increase in a four-year period—the rural–urban differential has not changed significantly.

Figure 3.1 graphically displays the pristine relationship between physician supply and population density. The physician supply is a linear function of population density; the more urban a county, the higher will be the relative physician supply. Physicians tend to settle in cities, and the current market does not reward rural practice.

Table 3.6 gives a more detailed picture of the location patterns of physicians with differing training and offers insight into the relative depletion of physicians in rural areas. General practitioners are more numerous in rural areas, yet hospital-based physicians and all other types of specialists work primarily in urban areas. In fact, most

TABLE 3.5. Active Nonfederal Physicians (MDs) per 10,000 Resident Population, According to Geographic Region and Location: United States, 1972 and 1976

| | All Regions | | Geographic Region | | | | | | | |
| | | | Northeast | | North Central | | South | | West | |
Location	1972	1976	1972	1976	1972	1976	1972	1976	1972	1976
Within SMSA	17.2	19.3	20.2	22.2	15.0	17.3	15.3	17.6	18.4	20.2
Outside SMSA	7.3	8.0	10.0	10.9	6.9	7.5	6.4	7.2	8.6	9.5
United States	14.5	16.2	18.8	20.6	12.5	14.2	12.0	13.8	16.4	17.9

Source: Adapted from *Health, United States, 1978,* DHEW Publication No. (PHS) 78–1232, December 1978, page 342, table 127.

TABLE 3.6. Patient-Care Physicians by Type of Practice per 10,000 Population, by Metropolitan–Nonmetropolitan Areas, 1979

| | Total in Patient Care | Office-Based Physicians | | | | Hospital-Based Practices |
		General Practice	Medical Specialties	Surgical Specialties	Other Specialties	
Total	15.39	2.10	3.02	3.50	2.62	4.16
SMSA	18.02	1.95	3.62	4.01	3.14	5.30
Non-SMSA	8.15	2.54	1.34	2.08	1.18	1.01

Source: Wunderman, Lorna E. *Physician Distribution and Medical Licensure in the U.S., 1979.* Chicago: American Medical Association, 1980.

TABLE 3.7. Physicians, Dentists, and Registered Nurses per 10,000 Resident Population, According to Geographic Region and Location: United States, Selected Years 1972–76

	Within SMSA	Outside SMSA	Overall
Active nonfederal physicians, 1976			
United States	19.3	8.0	16.2
Northeast	22.2	10.9	20.6
North Central	17.3	7.5	14.2
South	17.6	7.2	13.8
West	20.2	9.5	17.9
Licensed dentists, 1974			
United States	6.0	3.7	5.4
Northeast	7.2	4.8	6.9
North Central	5.6	4.2	5.2
South	4.8	2.8	4.1
West	6.9	4.8	6.5
Registered nurses employed in nursing, 1972			
United States	38.0	27.0	38.2
Northeast	46.7	47.7	51.4
North Central	36.7	29.6	38.4
South	32.2	18.7	28.8
West	35.3	28.8	36.5

Source: Adapted from *Health, United States, 1978*, DHEW Publication No. (PHS) 78–1232, December 1978, pages 344–346, Table 129.

general practitioners in rural areas are the survivors of an era that has passed, although the recent creation of the discipline of family medicine is beginning to increase their ranks. The great majority of physicians over the last several decades has chosen to specialize in increasingly narrow clinical disciplines, may be a pattern that is only now beginning to change. The way medical care is organized and produced has changed radically. Although the physician remains at the center of the medical sphere, the circumference has widened to include a wide spectrum of additional ancillary personnel, complex technology, and massive capital plants.[7] Until very recently, physicians have chosen to manage the increasing complexity of the medical world by

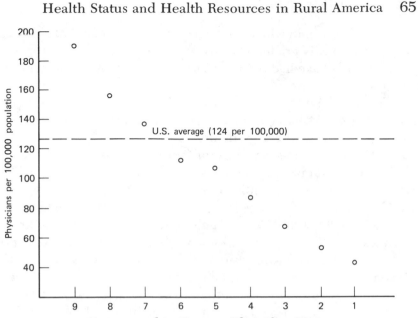

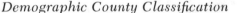

Demographic County Classification

1 - Nonmetropolitan counties with 0 to 9,999 inhabitants
2 - Nonmetropolitan counties with 10,000 to 24,999 inhabitants
3 - Nonmetropolitan counties with 25,000 to 49,999 inhabitants
4 - Nonmetropolitan counties with 50,000 or more inhabitants
5 - Counties considered potential SMSAs
6 - Counties in SMSAs with 50,000 to 499,999 inhabitants
7 - Counties in SMSAs with 500,000 to 999,999 inhabitants
8 - Counties in SMSAs with 1,000,000 to 4,999,999 inhabitants
9 - Counties in SMSAs with 5,000,000 or more inhabitants

Figure 3.1. Nonfederal physicians in the United States in direct patient care per 100,000 population, by county, from most urban (9) to most rural (1), in 1970. (Coleman, Sinclair. Physician Distribution and Rural Access to Medical Services. Santa Monica: Rand Corporation (R–1887), 1976.)

mastering smaller and smaller fragments of the whole. This progressive subdivision has created a situation in which an individual physician depends on the skills of a wide variety of others to operate effectively, must be backed up by a sophisticated technical plant, and requires a broad population base to generate sufficient patient demand to support increasingly narrow clinical spectra. This has promoted a situation in which specialists seek out urban areas. Since the majority of newly graduating physicians enter specialties, rural areas until recently have had no physician source to replace the generation of aging general practitioners who have been the mainstay of rural medical care. Physicians in rural areas are older than their urban counterparts, work longer hours, and earn less money, a situation not likely to entice younger graduates to join them.[8,9]

The issue of physician location is complex, and recent changes in the aggregate supply of physicians and the creation of the specialty in breadth called family medicine have begun to reverse some of the trends that are encapsulated in the preceding tables.[10] These issues will be discusssed more thoroughly in the next chapter and are central to some of the interventions needed to ensure an appropriate and equitable health care system for rural America. However, at the current time, physicians are underrepresented in rural America, and particularly with regard to specialized services or complex illnesses, rural dwellers are forced to travel to obtain medical care. Those physicians who do settle in rural areas seek out situations with preexisting medical practices, hospitals, and a more affluent economic base.[11] As Figure 3.1 demonstrates, the smaller and more remote the rural area, the less likely it is to have any residual medical care.

The sensitivity of other health providers to residential location mirrors that of physicians, although the effect is attenuated. As Table 3.7 shows, dentists also favor urban practice. Dentistry differs from medicine in that most dentists work in solo practice and are small entrepreneurs who are capable of working independently, requiring neither hospital facilities nor extensive support systems. Although dental equipment is costly, the capital investment is usually manageable, and most newly graduating dentists elect not to join existing group practices. Despite these economic factors, which would appear to permit dentists to establish successful practices in rural areas, dentists tend to locate in cities. This underlines the importance of social and professional factors in determining ultimate locations and the impact of the superior socioeconomic status and third-party coverage of urban dwellers in attracting and supporting health professionals.

Nursing personnel are also underrepresented in rural areas, although the differences are less dramatic than for physicians and dentists and are nonexistent in the northeastern United States. There are more than three times as many working nurses as physicians in rural areas, and in many cases they may substitute for physicians in patient care. This is true not only in the explicit curative functions of the newly created category of nurse practitioner, but also in the fact that nurses in rural hospitals have greater responsibilities and autonomy, often staffing emergency rooms and performing initial triage as well as definitive therapy for a number of conditions not traditionally considered within their professional purview.

Rural hospitals have recently experienced growing difficulty in obtaining adequate nursing personnel, particularly nurses both capable and willing to take on the diverse and often complex tasks required in the rural hospital setting. Although a great many nurses have been trained in our society, only 73 percent participate in the labor force.[12] Moreover, nurses tend to be relatively immobile and are willing to forego salary and other incentives so as not to move to new areas where their services are more in demand. New methods are needed to tap this important pool of manpower and to ensure that their skills are appropriate to the changing technological configurations of rural hospitals.

The flexibility of ancillary medical personnel, as well as the reservoir of medical paraprofessionals trained in a variety of settings ranging from the armed forces to fire departments, has led to the creation of a significant number of new health practitioners. This category encompasses not only nurse practitioners, but physician's assistants and Medex, who in general do not come from a formal nursing background. Many new health practitioner training programs were designed explicitly to train assistants to rural physicians and have measured their success against the extent to which their graduates have settled in rural areas.[13] At least for physician's assistants and Medex, as Table 3.8 and Figure 3.2 show, this experiment has been partially successful. In a 1975 survey of 685 active graduates of a variety of physician's assistant programs, 31 percent were practicing in towns of fewer than 10,000 people, which appears to reflect a tendency of these personnel to enter rural practice. On the other hand, graduate level nurse practitioners have remained largely in urban areas. The problems and prospects of using midlevel personnel in rural settings as physician extenders or physician substitutes is explored more fully in Chapter 4.

TABLE 3.8. Graduates of Physician Assistant Programs by Type of Practice as a Function of Size of Community in Which Practicing, 1975

Type of Practice	Under 10,000		10,000– 19,999		Size of Community 20,000– 49,999		50,000– 99,999		Over 100,000		Totals
	No.	%	No.	%	No.	%	No.	%	No.	%	Totals
Family practice	177	83	72	75	44	49	28	37	64	31	385
General internal medicine	9	5	8	8	20	22	6	8	31	15	74
Emergency medicine	7	3	4	4	3	3	4	5	25	12	43
General surgery	6	3	3	3	9	10	7	9	9	4	34
General pediatrics	3	1	—	—	2	2	3	4	12	6	20
Administrative	5	2	—	—	1	1	4	5	25	12	35
Other	6	3	10	10	12	13	24	32	42	20	94
Totals	213	100	97	100	91	100	76	100	208	100	685

Source: Donald W. Fisher, Physician Assistant: A Profile of the Profession, in: Hiestand DL, Ostow M (eds), *Health Manpower Information for Policy Guidance*. Cambridge, Mass, Ballinger Publishing Company, 1976, page 80, Table 7.2.

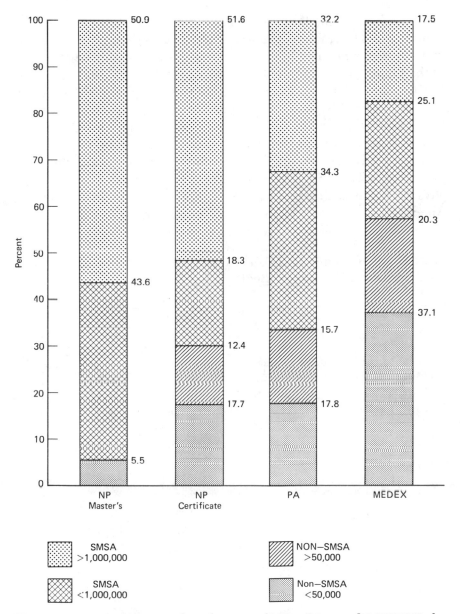

Figure 3.2. Employment distribution of NPs, PAs, and MEDEXs by county demographic area. (Figure 11-1, Nurse Practitioner and Physician Assistant Training and Deployment, DHEW Pub. No. (HRA) 77–3173, May 1977, page 18.)

The modern medical system has two major interlocking components: ambulatory and inpatient care. The economic relationship between these two essential parts of the system is somewhat unique to the United States. While ambulatory practices are established and run for the most part as small businesses by physicians acting as entrepreneurs, hospitals in general are not-for-profit institutions, either extensions of official governmental entities or quasi-public corporations owned and operated by nonprofit community boards. When we look at the supply of hospital beds in rural America—presented in Table 3.9—we confront an apparent paradox. Although physicians are scarce in rural areas, hospital beds are not. Rural America has *more* hospitals for its population than does urban

TABLE 3.9. Community Hospitals, According to Selected Characteristics, Geographic Regions, and Locations of Hospital: United States, 1976

	Within SMSA	Outside SMSA	Overall
Beds per 1,000 resident population			
United States	4.6	4.3	4.5
Northeast	4.5	4.3	4.5
North Central	5.1	4.9	5.0
South	4.8	4.2	4.6
West	3.8	3.7	3.8
Occupancy rate (%)			
United States	76.3	67.4	73.9
Northeast	81.8	75.8	81.0
North Central	78.1	66.4	74.5
South	74.1	67.9	72.0
West	67.9	59.8	66.3
Average number of beds per hospital			
United States	237	84	161
Northeast	275	129	238
North Central	282	86	166
South	217	83	141
West	179	61	128

Source: Adapted from *Health, USA, 1978*, DHEW Publication No. (PHS) 78–1232, December 1978, pages 368 and 369, Table 139.

America, and although these hospitals are considerably smaller, the number of beds available per 1,000 population does not differ greatly between the two demographic segments of the country. We explore the phenomenon of the rural hospital in detail in Chapter 6; suffice it to say that rural hospitals are well dispersed throughout the country. The challenge is not to create new rural hospitals but to use existing facilities appropriately within the context of a rationally designed health care system.[14]

The supply of medical services is one part of the equation that determines the ultimate level of utilization. People must be able to purchase the services rendered, especially in a system where almost all services are provided by private parties on a fee-for-service basis. Partially as a result of this, the medical care marketplace is dominated by third-party insurance. Most Americans are at least partially insulated from the full impact of medical bills by some insurance coverage on their behalf.

However, third-party coverage is erratic, and rural dwellers find themselves at a relative disadvantage in their ability to secure adequate insurance coverage. Since many of the best insurance plans are generated on the behalf of workers in large industries—and since large industries are infrequent in rural America—rural residents are both less likely to be covered by private insurance and more likely to have spotty coverage when they do obtain insurance.[15]

It might be expected that federal programs such as Medicare and Medicaid—aimed at the elderly and the poor, respectively—would take up some of the slack. This would be particularly logical in view of the observation that rural areas have a disproportionate percentage of the old and impoverished. However, the converse appears to be true. In studies by Davis and Marshall, the authors conclude that the current federal reimbursement programs systematically discriminate against rural dwellers and act as impediments to a more equitable distribution of medical services.[16] This is reflected in Tables 3.10 and 3.11, which demonstrate the dramatically diminished flow of federal funds to rural dwellers, despite their theoretical eligibility for these benefits. In addition, as Table 3.12 illustrates, voluntary insurance is also less prevalent in rural areas, particularly among farming families. Out-of-pocket expenditures constitute a large proportion of the medical budget for rural residents in general.

The problem is multifaceted. First, having a source of insurance

TABLE 3.10. Mean Expenditure for All Personal Health Services per Low Income Person[a] by Age and Residence, 1970

	Medicaid and Other Free Care			Percent of Expenditures Paid by Medicaid or Free Care		
Age	Rural	SMSA Central City	Other Urban	Rural	SMSA Central City	Other Urban
Birth to 17	$ 5	$ 76	$58	10.9	75.2	46.8
18 to 64	$52	$158	$83	32.9	43.9	23.6
65 and over	$27	$ 54	$38	6.6	12.1	11.6

Source: Ronald Andersen et al, *Expenditures for Personal Health Services: National Trends and Variations, 1953-1970.* U.S. Department of Health, Education, and Welfare, Health Resources Administration, October 1973.
[a]Low income defined as family income below $6,000.

is of little use if there are no physicians providing the insured service. A poor or elderly rural person may not have access to a physician and, with the paucity of transportation systems in rural areas, may be unable to travel to another community to seek services. The maldistribution of health personnel deprives rural dwellers of benefits otherwise available to them. Secondly, fee schedules are lower in rural areas; since programs such as Medicare pay on the basis of "usual and customary" charges, rural physicians receive less federal reimbursement for providing equivalent services. This has the effect of decreasing the effective demand for services in rural areas. If the

TABLE 3.11. Medicare Reimbursement per Enrollee in the U.S. by Metropolitan and Nonmetropolitan Residence, 1971

	All Medicare Benefits	Hospital and Posthospital Services	Physician and Other Medical Services
United States	357	262	100
SMSA	395	287	114
Non-SMSA	280	212	73

Source: U.S. Department of Health, Education, and Welfare, Social Security Administration, Office of Research and Statistics: *Medicare 1971, Reimbursement by State and County.* DHEW Pub. No. (SSA) 73–11704.

TABLE 3.12. Estimated Expenditures for All Personal Health Services by Residential Characteristics and Source of Payment: 1970

Residence	Source of Payment					Total Mean Expenditures per Person
	Medicaid, Welfare, Free Institution	Medicare	Voluntary Insurance	Out of Pocket		
SMSA, central city	30	21	73	99		235
SMSA, other	61	22	101	145		342
Urban, non-SMSA	16	17	57	94		190
Rural, nonfarm	12	18	70	93		199
Rural, farm	11	29	44	86		181

Source: Adapted from *Health of the Disadvantaged Chart Book.* DHEW Pub. No. (HRA) 77–628, 1977, page 97, Table 45.

intent of the federal programs was to ensure equity in access, it would be more logical to increase the reimbursement levels for rural providers, thus establishing an economic base that would tend to draw physicians from the cities. However, with the current reimbursement structure, the converse prevails.[17]

Actual utilization of health services is a function of several factors: need, as measured by health status and the sociodemographic composition of the population; available resources, as measured by the supply of health providers and facilities; and financial capability to purchase services, as reflected in relative economic status and the scope of third-party coverage. The utilization figures in Table 3.13 for doctors, dentists, and short-stay general hospitals support the contention that, of all these forces, utilization is most sensitive to supply. Rural dwellers see physicians and dentists less frequently than do people who live in metropolitan areas, either in central cities or the suburban fringe. These data have been corroborated in a later study by Aday and coworkers who observed that rural people had many fewer visits per year to physicians and dentists than their urban counterparts.[18] However, rural dwellers are more likely to have a hospitalization during the course of the year. This latter observation has a number of possible explanations. Hospital use may be determined by the relative supply; since rural areas are well supplied with hospital beds, there may be a tendency on the part of physicians to fill them in order to maintain the fiscal integrity of rural hospitals. A second plausible explanation is that there is a substitution effect. Over-worked rural physicians tend to use hospitals to extend their effectiveness; complex or severely ill patients who might be managed on an ambulatory basis in an urban area are hospitalized in a rural area because the physician with a crowded office cannot find time during the course of a routine day to resolve their problems. The rural hospital becomes an extension of the doctor's office, a flexible reservoir that can absorb unanticipated overflow in the work load. A third explanation is that rural dwellers are sicker when they present themselves to physicians and are, thus, more likely to be hospitalized.

Figure 3.3 takes a closer look at rural physician utilization. As we noted earlier, changes in the way medical care is produced and in the reward and value structure of the medical profession has caused a dichotomy in physician settlement patterns. Whereas the majority of

TABLE 3.13. Age-Adjusted Number of Physician Visits, Dental Visits, and Short-Stay Hospital Discharges per Person per Year, by Geographic Region: United States, 1973, 1974

| | | SMSA | | |
	All Areas	Central City	Noncentral City	Non-SMSA
Physician visits				
All regions	5.0	5.2	5.2	4.4
Northeast	5.0	5.4	4.9	4.3
North Central	4.9	5.1	5.3	4.3
South	4.8	4.8	5.1	4.5
West	5.4	5.8	5.7	4.5
Dental visits				
All regions	1.6	1.6	1.9	1.3
Northeast	2.0	2.0	2.1	1.6
North Central	1.6	1.5	1.8	1.4
South	1.3	1.3	1.6	1.1
West	1.9	1.8	2.1	1.6
Short-stay hospital discharges				
All regions	.141	.135	.129	.160
Northeast	.123	.126	.112	.144
North Central	.148	.152	.136	.159
South	.153	.136	.143	.172
West	.130	.122	.129	.144

Source: U.S. Department of Health, Education, and Welfare, National Center for Health Statistics, unpublished tabulations.

physicians in metropolitan areas are specialists, the converse is true in nonmetropolitan areas. Since few specialists practice in rural areas and the aggregate supply of physicians in rural America is relatively low, patients have longer waits and shorter visits in the offices of rural physicians. And since, until recently, the stock of rural general practitioners was the residue of professionals trained in another era, it might be expected that rural dwellers do not have the advantage of recent changes in the technology of medical care.

The evidence presented in this chapter supports the contention

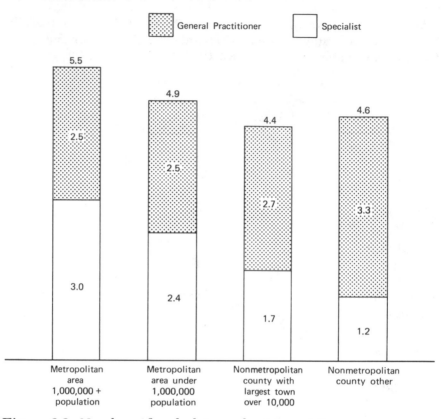

Figure 3.3. Number of ambulatory physician visits per person per year by type of physician and place of residence, 1973.

that rural Americans have difficulty obtaining health services. The major cause of this difficulty is the propensity of physicians—accelerated over the last several decades—to locate in cities. Physicians in rural areas are the stubborn remnants of an era that has passed, and it will require more time before recently graduated family physicians are available in sufficient numbers to replace their general practice predecessors.

The settlement pattern of physicians has important consequences for the other components of the health care system. Hospitals depend on physicians for their existence, and other health care institutions, such as nursing homes and public health departments, cannot run in an entirely autonomous fashion. The deficiency of health professionals in rural areas makes it difficult for rural dwellers to gain access to health care services, a fact reflected in their lower utilization rates.

The problem is exacerbated by the difficulty of paying for health services in rural areas. Rural dwellers tend to be poorer and older than their urban counterparts, but both private and public insurance programs are deficient in rural America. This lack of insurance tends to perpetuate a vicious cycle, undermining the economic base that physicians seek when deciding to establish new practices.

It is not clear whether it is healthier to live and work in rural areas. However, since rural areas tend to be reservoirs of the poor and elderly, as well as disadvantaged minority groups, the need for health care is higher in rural America despite the deficient resources. This disjunction between need and supply is a major challenge to the creation of workable, accessible rural health care systems.

REFERENCES

1. Balinsky W, Berger R: A review of the research on general health status indexes. *Medical Care* 13:283–293, 1975.
2. Diehr PK, Richardson WC, Shortell SM, LoGerfo JP: Increased access to medical care: The impact on health. *Medical Care* 17:989–999, 1979.
3. McCoy JL, Brown DL: Survey of low-income aged and disabled. *Social Security Bulletin* 41:14–26, 1978.
4. Matthews TH: *Health services in rural America.* Agricultural Information Bulletin No. 362, USDA. 1974.
5. Martin E: The federal initiative in rural health. *Public Health Reports* 90:291–297, 1975.
6. Andersen R, Kravits J, Anderson O: *Equity in Health Services: Empirical Analysis in Social Policy.* Cambridge, Mass, Ballinger, 1975.
7. Rushmer RF: *National Priorities for Health: Past, Present, and Projected.* New York, John Wiley and Sons, 1980.
8. *Profile of Medical Practice.* Chicago, American Medical Association, Center for Health Services Research and Development, 1974.
9. Thorndike N: 1975 net incomes and work patterns of physicians in five medical specialties. *Research and Statistics Note 13*, SSA, US-DHEW, July 21, 1977.
10. Geyman JP: *Family Practice: Foundation of Changing Health Care.* New York, Appleton-Century-Crofts, 1980.
11. Cotterill PG, Eisenberg BS: Improving access to medical care in underserved areas: The role of group practice. *Inquiry* 10:141–153, 1979.

12. Fagin C: The shortage of nurses in the United States. *Journal of Public Health Policy,* 293–311, 1980.
13. Scheffler RM: *The supply and demand for new health professionals: Physicians assistants and Medex.* Final report submitted to USDHEW, contract 1–44184. November 1977.
14. Rosenblatt RA: Planning ensures local and referral care for remote rural areas. *Hospitals* 53:83–88, 1979.
15. Ahearn MC: Health care in rural America. *Agricultural Information Bulletin No. 428,* USDA. 1979.
16. Davis K, Marshall R: *Primary Health Care Services for Medically Underserved Populations.* Papers on the National Health Guidelines: The priorities of Section 1502. USDHEW, DHEW Publication No. (HRA) 77–641. January 1977, p 1–31.
17. Davis K, Marshall R: New developments in the market for rural health care in Scheffler R (ed): Research in Health Economics, Volume I. Greenwich, Conn, JAI Press, 1979.
18. Aday L, Andersen R, Fleming G: *Health Care in the U.S.: Equitable for Whom?* Beverly Hills, Calif, Sage Publications, 1980.

CHAPTER 4

Primary Care:
The Foundation
of the Rural Health
Care System

*"It has been said that good medicine is many ordinary things
done well."*[1]

The delivery of primary care is the foundation of the rural health care
system. Primary care represents the first level of personal health
services.[2] It is the entry point to the health care system for most
people. There is not at present a clear and widely accepted definition
of primary care. The recent Institute of Medicine (IOM) study of
primary care manpower policy identified 38 definitions of primary
care that are currently being used.[2] Primary care has been defined
alternatively by the disciplinary training of providers, by the scope of
services provided, by the location of care, by the attributes of the
medical care process, and by the characteristics of encounters with
providers.

For our purpose, primary care can be defined as the level of
entry into the health care system where basic medical services are
provided. It includes the diagnosis and treatment of common illness
and disease, preventive services, home care services, and uncomplicated minor surgery and emergency care.[3,4] This definition brings

into focus the crucial issue of the relationship of the delivery of primary care to the total health care system. The IOM study concluded that integration of services should be one of the bases of a definition of primary care. Figure 4.1 depicts an idealized three-tiered health care system with primary care representing the entry level to the system and illustrates linkages among the primary, secondary, and tertiary care sectors.

This chapter will focus on the provision of primary care by rural health providers and the receipt of primary care by rural health consumers, with special attention paid to the relationships that exist between rural health systems and rural primary care. There are no simple answers to the question of how rural primary care can be most effectively provided. Despite the simplistic notion that most rural health problems can be solved by the presence of a physician in town, it has become clear that a variety of solutions is required to meet the primary care needs of diverse rural communities.[5]

A functioning health care system is required to make rural life viable.[6] Within the health care sector, the delivery of primary care has a significant role. Recent health planning legislation (Section 1502 of PL 93–641, the National Health Planning and Resources Development Act) has identified the provision of primary care services for medically underserved populations, particularly those located in rural or economically depressed areas, as the number one national health priority.[7] This priority will most likely receive increased attention as shifting demographic trends contribute to a growing rural population with "the people left behind being joined by those who changed their minds."[8]

RURAL PRIMARY CARE—A COMMUNITY PERSPECTIVE

THE AVAILABILITY AND ACCESSIBILITY OF RURAL PRIMARY CARE

From a community perspective, the availability and accessibility of primary health care providers is a major concern. The availability of rural primary health care providers refers to the sheer physical

**TERTIARY MEDICAL CARE AND HEALTH SERVICES:
FOR A STATE OR MULTIPLE COUNTY REGION**

(Provided in a Medical Center of
a University Teaching Center)

Quality specialty care in a personalized fashion:

1. Specialized medical, diagnostic, and therapeutic services for unusual and complicated cases.
2. Specialized surgical care for unusual and complicated cases (neurosurgery, organ transplants, etc.)
3. Specialized dental care for unusual and complicated oral disease and surgery.
4. Emergency medical care.
5. Part of a comprehensive health care system.

**SECONDARY MEDICAL CARE AND HEALTH SERVICES:
FOR A REGION**

(Provided in a Regional Hospital or Health Center)

Quality secondary and referral care in an available and personalized fashion:

1. Medical and surgical diagnostic services for complicated problems.
2. Surgical care and medical care for complicated problems.
3. Services for major surgical and medical emergency problems.
4. Specialty dental care—orthodontics, endodontics, periodontics.
5. Emergency medical care.
6. Part of a comprehensive health care system.

**PRIMARY MEDICAL CARE AND HEALTH SERVICES:
FOR AN AREA**

(Provided in an Area Health Ambulatory Center)

Quality primary care and health services in an available, personalized, and continuous fashion:

1. Preventive services, case-finding services, and diagnosis and treatment for usual and uncomplicated illness and disease.
2. Minor surgery and medical care for uncomplicated problems.
3. Home care programs—nursing services.
4. Preventive, diagnostic, and restorative dental services.
5. Part of a comprehensive health care system.
6. (In large Area Health Centers, services for surgical and medical problems not requiring specialized personnel and equipment.)

(Provided in a Community Health Center, usually a satellite to
an Area Primary Health Center)

Quality primary medical care and health services in an available, personalized, and continuous fashion:

1. Preventive services, case-finding services, and diagnosis and treatment for usual and uncomplicated illness and disease.
2. Supervision of home care health services.
3. Part of the comprehensive health care system.

Figure 4.1. A stratified health system. (Bureau of Community Health Services: Building a Rural Health System. USDHEW, 1976.)

presence in rural areas of health professionals able to care for the basic health care needs of the rural populace. There has been a significant increase in the supply of health professionals during the last few decades, largely due to policies developed in response to perceived shortages in the early 1960s. Table 4.1 presents trends and projections for the supply of physicians, dentists, and registered nurses over the 30-year period 1960–90. For the period 1960–75, there have been increases of almost 50 percent in the number of physicians, 25 percent in the number of dentists, and 80 percent in the number of registered nurses. These gains in the supply of health professionals can be traced to legislation that stimulated a dramatic increase in the annual number of graduates from health professional schools. Even more striking are the projected increases of almost 60 percent in the number of physicians, 35 percent in the number of dentists, and 75 percent in the number of registered nurses for the period 1975–90. These projections have led many to warn of an imminent oversupply of health professionals, particularly physicians, in the not too distant future.[9]

What have been the implications of this dramatic increase in the supply of health professionals on the number and location of primary health care providers? Table 4.2 presents a breakdown for selected years of the number and percent of physicians by specialty group. The significant increases in the supply of physicians, both actual and projected, have not been accompanied by major changes in the proportion of physicians in primary care specialties. In fact, we have seen a small decrease over the past 20 years in the proportion of physicians in primary care specialties. It is anticipated that shifts in the distribution of available residency slots will raise this proportion over the next decade to a point comparable to that which existed in the early 1960s.

Table 4.3 presents data on the distribution over time of the number of nonfederal physicians providing patient care. It is obvious that the increase in physician supply has not been shared equally by metropolitan and nonmetropolitan counties. In fact, nonmetropolitan counties have had a steadily declining percentage of all physicians locating within their boundaries. There is, however, significant variation by specialty of the distribution of physicians, as can be seen in Table 4.4. The lack of specialists in rural areas is apparent, but general practitioners are distributed considerably more evenly, with

TABLE 4.1. Health Manpower Supply: Trends and Projections

| Discipline | Year | Supply | | Professional to Population Ratio |
		Number (Thousands)	Professionals per 100,000 Population	
Physicians (MDs and DOs)	1960	259.5	143.6	1:696
	1970	323.2	157.8	1:634
	1975	378.6	177.3	1:564
	1980	444.0	199.3	1:502
	1985	519.0	221.7	1:451
	1990	594.0	242.4	1:413
Dentists	1960	90.1	49.4	1:2,024
	1970	102.3	49.6	1:2,016
	1975	112.8	52.9	1:1,890
	1980	127.0	57.1	1:1,751
	1985	141.7	60.5	1:1,653
	1990	153.0	62.4	1:1,603
Registered nurses	1960	504.0	282.0	1:355
	1970	722.0	356.0	1:281
	1975	906.0	427.0	1:234
	1980	1,152.0	520.0	1:192
	1985	1,345.0–1,380.0	579.0–584.0	1:171–1:173
	1990	1,484.0–1,587.0	616.0–653.0	1:153–1:162

Source: Scheffler R, et al: Physicians and new health practitioners: Issues for the 1980's. *Inquiry* 16:195–229, 1979, Table 1.

TABLE 4.2. Number of Active Physicians (MDs) and Percentage Distribution by Specialty Groups

Specialty	1963		1968		1976		1980[b]		1990[b]	
	Number	Percent	Number	Percent	Number	Percent	Number	Percent	Number	Percent
All specialties	261,728	100.0	296,312	100.0	348,443	100.0	430,150	100.0	566,930	100.0
Primary care specialties[a]	110,071	42.1	116,760	39.4	135,881	39.0	166,790	38.8	239,830	42.3
Other medical specialties	12,291	4.7	15,762	5.3	18,955	5.4	26,580	6.2	41,080	7.2
Surgical specialties	67,745	25.8	81,820	27.6	98,667	28.3	113,200	26.3	129,610	22.9
All other specialties	71,621	27.4	81,970	27.7	94,940	27.3	123,580	28.4	156,410	27.6

Source: Scheffler R, et al: Physicians and new health practitioners: Issues for the 1980's. *Inquiry* 16:195–229, 1979, Table 2, and Interim Report of the Graduate Medical Education National Advisory Committee to the Secretary, DHHS, 1978, Table 14.

[a]Includes general practice, family practice, general internal medicine, and general pediatrics.
[b]Projections.

TABLE 4.3. Nonfederal Physicians (MDs) Providing Patient Care in Metropolitan and Nonmetropolitan Areas, 1963–76

| | | Percent and Number of MDs per 100,000 Population | | | |
| | | Metropolitan | | Nonmetropolitan | |
Year	All Counties	Number	Percent	Number	Percent
1963	120.3	144.2	79.1	73.8	20.9
1964	122.0	146.8	79.4	73.9	20.6
1965	123.2	148.7	79.7	73.6	20.3
1966	123.7	148.9	79.9	74.1	20.1
1967	125.4	150.0	81.2	73.3	18.8
1968[a]	118.7	141.6	81.3	69.7	18.7
1969	121.8	145.7	81.6	70.5	18.4
1970	124.2	148.7	81.8	71.5	18.2
1971	127.5	152.9	83.1	70.1	16.9
1972	128.5	152.9	84.6	68.6	15.4
1973	129.1	150.9	85.6	69.4	14.4
1974	130.9	153.3	85.5	70.4	14.5
1975	134.8	156.9	86.6	74.1	13.4
1976	137.4	158.2	86.6	74.4	13.4

Source: Interim Report of the Graduate Medical Education National Advisory Committee to the Secretary, *DHHS*, 1978, Table 13.

[a]Beginning in 1968, the AMA changed its methods of classifying physicians to reflect the number of hours spent in various activities and specialties. This resulted in a loss of physicians in patient care with corresponding increases in "other activities" and inactive.

rural areas actually having a higher ratio of general practitioners to population than metropolitan areas. This trend continues, as over one-half of the graduating residents in family practice currently enter practice in communities with populations of less than 25,000.[10]

There presently appears to be an adequate overall supply of physicians in the United States, but problems of geographic and specialty distribution persist.[2] We are producing increasing numbers of primary care physicians but at the same time churning out an oversupply of specialists. Despite the encouraging proportion of family practice residency graduates entering rural practice, there still is a serious geographic maldistribution of health providers in our country. The increased morbidity of rural populations, as well as the advanced age of rural physicians, suggests that we will continue to need more rural primary care practitioners.[11]

TABLE 4.4. Physicians in Patient Care per 100,000 Population by Type of Practice and Residence, 1975

Residence	General Practitioners	Office Based		Other Specialists
		Medical Specialists	Surgical Specialists	
Metropolitan	19.9	30.9	36.3	25.6
Greater	20.4	35.5	37.7	29.0
Core	21.7	39.3	41.9	32.2
Fringe	17.4	27.0	28.4	21.8
Medium	19.5	25.4	34.3	21.3
Lesser	18.7	24.1	34.7	21.6
Nonmetropolitan	25.9	10.5	18.3	9.2
Urbanized				
Adjacent to SMSA	22.9	15.5	25.7	13.0
Nonadjacent to SMSA	21.6	19.7	33.9	17.7
Less Urbanized				
Adjacent to SMSA	27.7	6.6	11.6	5.6
Nonadjacent to SMSA	29.9	7.7	15.2	7.4
Total Rural				
Adjacent to SMSA	25.3	1.7	3.5	1.8
Nonadjacent to SMSA	26.1	2.9	4.5	2.7
U.S. total	21.5	25.3	31.4	21.2

Source: Ahearn M: Health Care in Rural America. Agriculture Information Bulletin No. 428, U.S. Department of Agriculture, July 1979, Table 7.

It is difficult to provide a convincing argument based on empirical evidence that any of the approaches used to alter the urban/rural distribution of health providers has had a significant impact.[12,13] Moreover, the findings of a recent study that suggests that market forces have started to cause sizable changes in the distribution of board-certified specialists are preliminary at best and misleading at worst.[14,15] The fact remains that many rural communities continue to have difficulty recruiting and retaining physicians and other health personnel for a myriad of well-documented reasons, including the lack of adequate facilities and resources, professional isolation, inadequate organizational frameworks, overwork, economic disincentives, excessive demands on the personal life of the provider, life style preferences, and spouse influence.[16] Those communities with the greatest need will continue to have the most trouble in attracting health care providers.[5]

The previous discussion concerned itself solely with the availability of primary health care resources in rural areas. The past decade, however, has seen tremendous interest focused on the accessibility of primary care services for the entire population with particular emphasis on underserved rural and inner-city areas. Accessibility refers to those characteristics of a health care system that hinder or aid the use of health care resources by a given population. The use of health services by a rural population is often related to factors other than the availability of health services in rural areas.[17] The list of barriers facing rural residents in their efforts to receive primary care services is formidable, and includes economic factors such as lower income levels and less comprehensive health insurance coverage; sociocultural factors relating to particular ethnic and/or racial attitudes and beliefs; limited health resources in rural areas resulting in longer travel distances and higher travel costs; and inadequate transportation and communication systems.[16]

In spite of the above, recent evidence suggests that there has been considerable improvement in access to health care services for most Americans, including rural residents. The Center for Health Administration Studies (CHAS) at the University of Chicago has completed health care surveys of a stratified sample of the United States population in 1963, 1970, and 1976. Their most recent findings indicate that every subpopulation that was studied, including rural farm and rural nonfarm, had better access to medical services in 1976 than in 1970 or 1963.[18] Table 4.5 presents data for

TABLE 4.5. Changes in Access to Health Care by Residence: 1970–76

		SMSA Central City	SMSA Other Urban	Non-SMSA Urban	Rural Nonfarm	Rural Farm	Total
Percent without regular source of care	1970	15	10	6	8	12	11
	1976	15	13	10	10	7	12
Percent with travel time to regular source more than 30 minutes	1970	10	8	8	12	25	11
	1976	7	7	5	12	15	9
Percent seeing a physician in year	1970	65	72	71	68	62	68
	1976	77	78	73	75	68	76

Source: Aday L, Andersen R, Fleming G: Health Care in the U.S.—Equitable for Whom? Beverly Hills, Calif. Sage Publications, 1980, Tables 2.1, 2.7, and 3.1.

1970 and 1976 on selected access indicators by residence. The rural farm population improved its access as measured by percent of the population with a regular source of care, percent who traveled less than 30 minutes to a regular source, and percent who saw a physician in the past year. The rural nonfarm population was more likely to have seen a physician in the past year, experienced no change in travel time measures, but had a slight increase in the percent of its members without a regular source of care.

The finding that rural access to health care has generally improved in recent years does not imply, however, that the access problem has been solved for rural Americans. Tables 4.6 through 4.8 present the most recent CHAS findings (1976) on a variety of access indicators by the location of residence. Rural subpopulations were more dissatisfied with the convenience and availability of health services, and saw health providers less frequently than their urban counterparts. In addition, rural farm residents were more likely to be uninsured or without comprehensive insurance coverage, with the latter observation reflected in Table 4.8 by the greater proportion of individual policies for the rural farm population.

There are still large groups of rural residents with special problems in gaining access to health care services. Among these groups are migrant farm workers, farm households in economically depressed areas, low income families not covered by group health insurance contracts, blacks in the rural South, and native Americans. Aday et al. suggest that any new initiatives that address remaining access problem areas must be well targeted to specific populations rather than comprehensive in nature.[18] There are no uniform answers to the access problems that continue to face rural dwellers. It is clear that simply attracting more physicians and other health personnel to rural areas is not always the solution. Readily accessible, newly started rural primary care practices are often not used due to the inertia encountered in overcoming previously established patterns of care of rural residents.[19]

The improvement over the past two decades in rural residents' access to health care services makes us optimistic about the future. However, barriers to further progress remain. Engrained in our current health care system are powerful disincentives to the effective training, placement, and use of primary health care professionals.

TABLE 4.6. Assessment of Access to Health Care According to Access Indicators by Selected Demographic Groups—1976

| | | | | | Blacks | |
	U.S. Population (%)	Suburban Resident (%)	Farm Resident (%)	Urban (%)	Rural South (%)
Access Indicators					
Regular Source of Care					
With	88	87	93	84	90
Without	12	13	7	16	10
Convenience					
Travel Time to Doctor					
15 minutes or less	48	51	27	40	38
More than 15 minutes	52	49	73	60	62
Waiting time in MD's office					
30 minutes or less	64	69	53	62	44
More than 30 minutes	36	31	47	38	56
Time spent with MD					
15 minutes or more	72	73	67	78	76
Less than 15 minutes	28	27	33	22	24
Utilization					
Seeing a doctor in past year					
Saw	76	78	68	77	65
Did not see	24	22	32	23	35
Seeing a dentist in past year					
Saw	49	52	45	39	18
Did not see	51	48	55	61	82

Source: Health Resources Administration: *Health of the Disadvantaged: Chart Book II.* DHHS, September 1980, Table 56.

TABLE 4.7. Percent More Dissatisfied than the Median Person in the National Population with Aspects of Medical Care by Residence—1976

Residence	Percent More Dissatisfied than Median				Sample Size
	Convenience of Services	Availability of Services	General Dissatisfaction		
SMSA central city	52	47	50		1,371
SMSA other urban	45	39	48		1,727
Non-SMSA urban	52	62	50		751
Rural nonfarm	54	66	55		1,018
Rural farm	54	60	51		268
Total	50	50	50		5,135

Source: Aday L, Andersen R, Fleming G: *Health Care in the U.S.—Equitable for Whom?* Beverly Hills, Calif, Sage Publications, 1980, Table 4.2.

TABLE 4.8. Residence of People Under 65 Years of Age with Selected Modes of Insurance Coverage—1976

| | Mode of Insurance Coverage | | | | |
	Group Policy (%)	Individual Policy (%)	Medicaid or Reduced Price Care (%)	Uninsured (%)	Distribution of Total Population (%)
Residence					
SMSA central city	24	22	39	30	26
SMSA other urban	39	34	29	32	37
Non-SMSA urban	12	10	11	9	12
Rural nonfarm	20	20	21	22	20
Rural farm	5	13	2	8	6

Source: Aday L, Andersen R, Fleming G: *Health Care in the U.S.—Equitable for Whom?* Beverly Hills, Sage Publications, 1980, Table 2.24.

Major technological advances have resulted in a medical education system that fosters the training of specialists and a reimbursement system that penalizes those who provide primary care services.[16] Ineffective local planning and lack of flexible organizational alternatives have hindered those dedicated to improving access to primary care services in rural areas. Even those programs designed for specific populations often must overcome major implementation barriers at the local level that arise from the need to balance political, fiscal, ethical, and legal concerns.[20]

But perhaps the largest obstacle to increased access to health care is the current emphasis on cost containment. Can we on the one hand develop standards that recommend primary care services be available within 30-minutes travel time and accessible on a 24-hour basis and on the other hand strive for reduced system-wide health care costs? There is no obvious answer to this question, but a broad systems approach rather than one that focuses on manpower or facilities or reimbursement is needed to increase access to primary care services in our present complex health care system.

COMMUNITY INVOLVEMENT WITH RURAL PRIMARY CARE

One of the primary attributes of a viable, self-sustaining rural primary care system is *community ownership*. By community ownership we are not necessarily referring to the legal ownership of a facility and/or equipment but rather the involvement of the community and its leaders in the planning, design, implementation, and maintenance of a system designed to provide primary care services for a rural population. This type of involvement has occurred too infrequently in the past and is a major explanation of the slow growth of new rural primary care practices, as consumers continue to use their previous physicians and bypass the newly established rural system. It is important that the individuals who are expected to use a primary health care system participate in its development. Unfortunately, most rural communities lack individuals with the expertise, both from an administrative and leadership perspective, to foster health care developmental activities.[21]

But the times are changing. Demographic shifts in recent years have led to an increase in rural population, both absolutely and relative to that of urban areas. These population shifts heighten the need for rationally planned rural health care systems and also increase the growing potential for the significant involvement of the rural populace in designing the social systems that it will use. Rural dwellers need to understand the significance of their role in the health care system, beyond that of simply being the consumers of health services.

Community Diagnosis.   The first step in community involvement with health care system development is self-diagnosis. Communities must be able to assess their needs for health care services and set priorities for unmet needs.[22] The irony is that those communities with the greatest needs are least likely to have the capability of assessing and setting priorities for those needs.[23]

Assessing the existence of unmet needs is by no means a trivial task. The U.S. General Accounting Office has criticized the National Health Service Corps for not adequately considering the potential demand for services when assessing physician need in health manpower shortage areas.[24] The Index of Medical Underservice, which has been used by the federal government as the basis for determining geographic areas that are medically underserved, has been criticized for not accounting for population needs and existing utilization patterns nor measuring the quality of existing resources.[5]

Needs assessment can be best accomplished locally. The individual rural citizen's perception of health needs is influenced by local social and economic conditions. Residents of a community are able to collect information on the demographic structure of their geographic area, the existing health problems of the population, and the utilization patterns that have developed in response to these problems.

There are other aspects of community diagnosis that are often overlooked but are just as important as health needs assessment. Not all communities can initiate new and creative rural health programs. A community must assess whether it has the necessary resources of leadership, administration, and fiscal support required for the development of innovative health programs. It must determine whether there is a readiness to act, whether there are leaders and constituents willing to cope with the uncertainty of change.[25] This is a critical task because opposition to change is often characteristic of rural areas.

The greater financial risk of capital investment in rural areas increases the need for a thorough understanding of the community's fiscal capability before the development of health programs. The rural tax base is relatively meager, and the sparseness of the population often limits the capability to support essential levels of health services.[26,27] Moreover, limited fiscal resources may force rural communities to make choices among better health care systems, improved roads, or improved educational systems. Communities need to assess the importance of health care in relationship to their other existing social and economic needs and determine whether they are willing to share the risk associated with the development of improved health care systems.

The self-sufficient rural community no longer exists. The complex task of improving rural social systems, including health care systems, requires an honest assessment of a rural community's needs and its capacity to meet those needs.

Community Involvement with the Planning Process.   To date, the health planning process has been largely insensitive to the needs of the rural populace. This insensitivity can be traced to the fact that most health planning has been initiated by governmental forces external to the local community. An excellent example of this point was the promulgation of the National Health Planning Guidelines that were discussed in Chapter 2.

With the uncertainty currently surrounding the existing federal health planning apparatus, rural communities have the opportunity to start planning for themselves. Effective local planning is a necessary ingredient for the future well-being of rural primary care delivery systems. It is necessary if rural health systems are to cope with stressful events, such as the retirement or death of a physician, the declining status of the local hospital, or the impact of population growth due to the boom town phenomenon.

Two central issues relating to community involvement with the planning process are (1) who will do the planning and, (2) what activities are involved in the planning process. Community sponsorship of rural health care system improvements starts with the self-diagnosis described earlier and includes the planning, implementation, and maintenance of system changes. Often this sponsorship comes from a nonprofit community group, such as the local hospital board. In many communities, the hospital board has a long-standing tradition of being the most influential local health policy-making group. However, one can appreciate the complex problem facing hospital board members who on the one hand are concerned with the fiscal stability of the local hospital and are also asked to plan for improved primary care services for the community.

At the other extreme, rural health care innovations can be the result of the concerted efforts of individual leaders rather than core groups.[28] Broader representation on sponsoring groups should, however, improve the acceptance and longevity of rural health system innovations. Whether the core group has one or 10 members, there is often a scarcity of individuals with leadership talent in rural areas. Rural communities have failed to develop leaders who are willing and able to accept public office.[29] This situation must change if effective rural sponsorship of health planning activities is to be accomplished.

The range of activities involved with the population-based planning of primary care services is extensive. The first step has already been described in the section on community diagnosis. Accurate assessment of community needs can be best accomplished at the local level. Needs assessment must be community based and requires an understanding of the demographic structure of the population, rational geographic boundaries for health service delivery, and knowledge of disease patterns in the target population and how they are handled.

Based on the above, estimates can be made of the gap between primary care services currently offered and those required for the population. Translation of needs for primary care services into new programs, personnel, and/or facilities is the next step in the planning process. Of initial importance is consideration of the trade-offs between short-term interventions (e.g., adding a physician, building a new clinic) and long-term development activities (e.g., increasing the industrial base in the community, improving sanitation, plumbing, and sewage systems).[30] Given the availability of federal funds, the short-term intervention strategy has been frequently attempted in many rural areas in our country, whereas long-term developmental activities have been more commonly used as a strategy for improving the delivery of primary care services in underdeveloped nations around the world. One particular problem with use of the latter approach in rural areas of our country has been the ineffectiveness of local governmental bodies in rural communities. Their lack of leadership and opposition to change has often frustrated long-range planning and developmental efforts.

A clear understanding of community goals and expectations for primary care services must also be developed.[31] Without knowing how a given population copes with the lack of health care services or its attitudes toward reasonable travel times, it is impossible to predict accurately how rapidly a new physician's practice will grow in that community. Unmet need must be translated into demand for services if new rural health programs are to become viable.

Having assessed community needs and expectations and evaluated the utility of short-term versus long-term planning strategies, local planners must address the issues of how the necessary primary care services will be provided. They must translate the need for services into personnel and facility requirements and associated financing strategies. Decisions must be made on the number and location of health providers necessary to deliver primary care services. This stage may include examining the feasibility of using non-physician personnel or the need for building a new clinic facility.

Solutions to the above questions are contingent on the ability to develop successful financing strategies for both the initial and operational phases of the project. Initial subsidies to offset capital outlays and start-up costs are often necessary for the development of new programs. In-kind contributions from the community in the form of donations or a rent-free facility can be very helpful. Of equal importance is the development of an ongoing fiscal plan resulting in long-term program financial viability. Identification of rural programs not capable of attaining self-sufficiency is important. Some rural areas will require ongoing assistance for their health programs due to an insufficient economic base in the community.[32]

Another essential part of the planning process consists of analysis of the linkages that must be developed between the local program and other resources, both inside and outside the local area. Rural health programs must be able to function within the context and constraints of the existing health care and governmental systems in the local area.[33] Young family physicians often have difficulty building new practices in rural areas dominated by older, well-established general practitioners.[34] The role of local government in the rural health care system must be explicitly considered. The range of possible activities for local government includes being the provider of services, reimburser of services, and/or planner and coordinator of services.[29] The breadth of the local government's role can be widened by pressures exerted by local citizenry committed to the importance of having an effective health care system.

The role of external forces on the local health care system can be considered from a variety of viewpoints. From a fiscal standpoint, external funds may be required to assure initial or ongoing viability. From a service delivery standpoint, health providers outside the local area may be the appropriate choice for the delivery of particular types of services. One would expect and hope that the overwhelming majority of primary care services would be delivered locally and external providers would be primarily involved with specialty referrals.

External forces can also act as catalysts of change in the local health care system.[30] This can be particularly advantageous for areas with limited resources and a lack of individuals with leadership and administrative talents. It can be troublesome, however, when change is accompanied by insensitive rules and regulations that ignore local needs.[35] To avoid this scenario, rural citizens need to participate in health policy development at the local, state, and federal levels. Although difficult and time consuming, this participation has recently been facilitated by the advent of several rural advocacy groups, including Rural America, the National Rural Center, the American Rural Health Association, and the National Rural Primary Care Association. These groups have the potential to strengthen the lobbying efforts on behalf of rural citizens in our country.

A final activity for local planners involves program maintenance. Once programs have been implemented, local involvement should not cease. We have already mentioned the critical importance of the development of realistic operational budgets to ensure financial self-sufficiency. Policy development and program accountability are two other areas in which ongoing community involvement is helpful. A community that has interest and monitors the performance and management of its health care programs will find its providers more responsive to local concerns.

Before concluding this section on community involvement with the planning process, we will describe an example of an organized attempt to incorporate community participation in the development of a rural health care system. Rural Health Associates (RHA) is a community-based, nonprofit corporation set up in 1971 to coordinate the development of a comprehensive primary care delivery system for the 30,000 residents of a 1,900 square mile area in west central Maine.[36] This corporation was established to facilitate the receipt of external support for the delivery of local health services, to activate and organize community forces in the local health care decision-making process, and to improve provider recruitment and the development of a comprehensive primary care delivery system.

Over the past decade, the efforts of Rural Health Associates have resulted in the development of a rural primary care group practice with 10 physicians and five mid-level practitioners, a health maintenance organization (HMO) for 3,000 low-income residents of the area, and several research and development activities. These accomplishments have not been achieved easily. From the outset, considerable opposition to Rural Health Associates was voiced by existing area health professionals. Public meetings did not help solve these problems. Moreover, disagreements with the local rural hospital administrative staff still persist and have resulted in a lack of necessary cooperation between this facility and RHA on such matters as the use of laboratory and x-ray facilities and the development of the HMO plan. Thus, even a well-planned endeavor with commitment to the development of a broad base of support can encounter community division over innovative plans to change the structure of the rural health care delivery system.

Summary.   Effective community involvement with the planning process starts with the diagnosis of community needs, expectations, and capabilities; translates those service needs into short- and long-term programs with associated personnel, facility, and economic requirements; examines the program linkages that must be developed with local government and external segments of the health care system; and concludes with continual involvement in program maintenance activities. In addition, participation in the development of health policy at all levels—local, state, and federal—is beneficial particularly with respect to the strengthening of lobbying efforts.

The exact nature and level of optimal community involvement naturally depends on the unique characteristics of the political, social, and economic structure of a particular rural community. There are no textbook solutions, but community involvement in the planning and development of rural health care systems should improve the long-run viability of these systems.

RURAL PRIMARY CARE—THE PROVIDER'S PERSPECTIVE

The shortage of qualified health personnel practicing in rural areas highlights the need for the optimal use of existing rural health providers. The traditional, solo, fee-for-service general practitioner has been unable to meet the primary care needs of the rural populace by himself. A variety of alternative approaches have sprouted in an attempt to fill the generalist role in the health care of rural families. This section will discuss private sector and alternative approaches to providing primary care services in rural areas.

THE RURAL PRIMARY CARE PHYSICIAN AS ENTREPRENEUR

On the Development of a Rural Primary Care Practice. The development of a rural primary care practice is a risky venture. From an economic perspective, fledgling rural primary care practices must be patient in their quest for financial stability. Even well-planned practices may require three years or more to alter the existing care-seeking patterns of a rural population.[34,37] Moreover, the development of a primary care practice requires that the physician become an entrepreneur. The physician must organize, manage, promote, and assume the risk of developing a rural practice. Table 4.9 lists the range of activities facing the initiator of a rural primary care practice. This list is formidable, particularly for one who has virtually no experience or formal training in many of these areas.

The new rural primary care practice is a fragile entity.[12] Well-established physicians often resent and resist the development of new primary care practices sponsored by physicians with backgrounds and ideas they view as unconventional.[38] The local hospital administrator may apply undue pressure on the young primary care physician if the administrator's expectations concerning the physician's use of the hospital are not met.[39] The patients of a new rural physician often want to "own, possess, love, and idealize the physician all at the same time."[40] It is a nontrivial task for the rural physician to balance his own needs against those of his patients, colleagues, and other health professionals involved with the delivery of rural primary care.

Madison has described the "small pond, big ripple" effect facing the rural medical practitioner.[12] The stability of a rural primary care practice is extremely dependent on the population and environment it serves. Changes in the social and economic structure of a small town can have a major impact on the emerging rural primary care practice. The closure of a factory with the associated emigration of workers and their families can destroy a rural medical practice. The ability to effectively adapt to environmental changes is essential to the long-term viability of rural primary care practice.

The Content of Rural Primary Care.   The role of the primary care physician in the rural health care system is still evolving. The well-trained family practitioner of today is capable of treating the majority of health care problems presented by a rural population. The family physician can provide definitive care for at least 95 percent of the patient care problems encountered in everyday medical practice.[10]

Table 4.10 presents the 20 most common diagnoses for office visits to United States physicians in 1979 as collected by the National Ambulatory Medical Care Survey (NAMCS). Visits associated with the top 20 diagnoses accounted for almost 40 percent of all visits to ambulatory care physicians with a wide range of acute (e.g., upper respiratory infection, otitis media, pharyngitis) and chronic diseases (e.g., hypertension, neurotic disorders, diabetes). In addition, normal pregnancy and health care of infants and children were the second and fifth most frequent diagnoses. Comparable results were also collected in the Virginia study, a two-year analysis of the health care problems that 88,000 patients presented to 118 family physicians located throughout the state of Virginia.[41] In this study, the top 20 diagnoses accounted for 48 percent of all problems seen by family physicians. The breakdown of the top 20 diagnoses was similar to the

TABLE 4.9. Guidelines for Designing Rural Community Practice Models

I. Background
   A. Planning
      1. Accessibility
         a. Personal
         b. Comprehensive
      2. Quality
         a. Professional
         b. Acceptability
         c. Standards
      3. Continuity
         a. Personal
         b. Central source–coordinated services
      4. Efficiency
         a. Administration
         b. Compensation
         c. Financing
   B. Recruitment
      1. Full-time staff
      2. Temporary staff
II. Organization design
   A. Nonprofit corporation
   B. Governing board
   C. Salaried professionals
   D. Management terms
   E. Linkages
III. Scope of services
   A. Comprehensive primary care
      1. Stratified patient care
   B. Referral system
      1. Two-tier system
   C. Specialty consultants
IV. Operational design
   A. Clinical programs
   B. Patient flow
   C. Medical records
   D. Medical audit
   E. Billing systems
   F. Outreach
      1. Preventive, supportive

TABLE 4.9. *(Continued)*

  G. Dentistry
  H. Pharmacology
  I.   Medical support services
  J.   Role of midlevel clinicians
  K. Family care units—hospital, clinic, home
  L. Education
        1. Inservice, continuing
 V. Finances
  A. Financial planning
        1. Short-term, long-term
  B. Identifying sources of support
        1. Grants, services
VI. Evaluation
  A. Identifying goals
        1. Operational objectives
  B. Measurement of goal attainment
  C. Management information system
        1. Manual versus computer
        2. Deficiencies and discrepancies
            a. Supply
            b. Demand
            c. Financing

Source: Stumbo W: Rural health centers and the development of progressive patient care. *Clinical Medicine* 84:10–13, 1979, Table 1.

NAMCS breakdown, with differences reflecting the type of problems (e.g., lacerations, abrasions, sprain and strains, abdominal pain) frequently seen by family physicians.

Rural primary care physicians have generally provided a wide range of health care services due to the lack of other health professionals in their locale. This includes the provision of hospital-based care by the rural primary care physician. The rural doctor has found the hospital to be a necessary resource from both a financial and clinical perspective. The contribution of hospital-based services to the physician's income and the desire to provide continuity of care between office-based and hospital-based services have led to an increasing role for the rural primary care physician in hospital care. The extent of the role, however, is dependent on the training and background of the physician as well as environmental factors, such

TABLE 4.10. Number and Percent of Office Visits, by the 20 Most Common Principal Diagnoses: United States, 1979

Rank	Most Common Principal Diagnosis	ICD–9–CM Code[a]	Number of Visits in Thousands	Percent of Visits
1	Essential hypertension	401	23,607	4.2
2	Normal pregnancy	V22	22,426	4.0
3	General medical examination	V70	16,575	3.0
4	Acute upper respiratory infections of multiple or unspecified sites	465	14,946	2.7
5	Health supervision of infant or child	V20	14,022	2.5
6	Suppurative and unspecified otitis media	382	11,166	2.0
7	Neurotic disorders	300	11,102	2.0
8	Allergic rhinitis	477	9,823	1.8
9	Diabetes mellitus	250	8,947	1.6
10	Disorders of refraction and accommodation	367	8,527	1.5

TABLE 4.10. (*Continued*)

11	Obesity and other hyperalimentation	278	8,348	1.5
12	Acute pharyngitis	462	8,149	1.5
13	Diseases of sebaseous glands	706	7,385	1.3
14	Special investigations and examina-			
	tions	V72	7,176	1.3
15	Follow-up examinations	V67	6,792	1.2
16	Asthma	493	6,786	1.2
17	Other forms of chronic ischemic			
	heart disease	414	5,857	1.1
18	Certain adverse effects not else-			
	where classified	995	5,697	1.0
19	Contact dermatitis and other eczema	692	5,683	1.0
20	Acute tonsilitis	463	5,420	1.0

Source: National Center for Health Statistics, March 1981.

*Based on International Classification of Diseases, Ninth Revision, Clinical Modification (ICD–9–CM).

as the availability of other physicians and community need.[42] The most frequent areas for hospital admissions for rural primary care physicians include obstetrical care, pediatric care, and geriatric care, with associated discharge diagnoses related to pregnancy, care of the newborn, and cardiovascular diseases.[42]

The granting of hospital privileges for rural primary care physicians is relatively straightforward; however, well-defined boundaries are usually established. In general, rural family practitioners have privileges in the obstetrical area, surgical area, the intensive care unit, and the coronary care unit.[43] The performance of surgery by rural primary care physicians is an example of the broad scope of services provided by many rural physicians. In 1976, the National Study on Surgical Services for the United States (SOSSUS) found that general practitioners represented 27 percent of all physicians who performed surgery but only nine percent of the total surgical workload.[44] Kane et al., however, found that one-fourth of the surgical procedures reimbursed by Blue Cross/Blue Shield in Utah were performed by general practitioners.[45] This expanded role of the primary care physician in the predominantly rural state of Utah reflects the impact of environmental factors on the role of the rural primary care physician.

The content of rural primary care is expanding. The older general practitioner who no longer practices obstetrics is being replaced by the younger family physician who wants hospital-based care to be an integral part of his practice. In turn, an aging population means that geriatric care will take an increasing proportion of the energies and time of the rural primary care physician. Barring major shifts in the distribution of medical specialists, rural primary care physicians will continue to play a broad role in patient care in the future.

The Organization of Rural Primary Care.   The rural physician faces a set of complex, interrelated organizational issues related to the development and maintenance of a primary care practice. This section will discuss two of these issues: (1) the choice of solo versus group practice and (2) the use of nonphysician personnel.

The Choice of Solo Versus Group Practice.   A major issue related to the development of a rural health care system is the organizational structure supporting the delivery of primary care services. The formation of group medical practices in rural areas has been championed as a means of improving the provision of rural primary care services both from an economic and quality-of-care perspective. Group medical practice may be defined as "three or more physicians organized to provide medical care through the joint use of equipment and personnel, with the income from the practice distributed according to a predetermined scheme and with services being rendered either on a fee-for-service basis or under some prepayment plan."[46]

Table 4.11 shows the steady growth of group practices throughout the United States for the 30-year period, 1946–75. The percent of rural physicians associated with group practices increased from 12 percent in 1960 to 20 percent in 1970.[47] Only 17 percent of recent family practice residents entered solo practice as compared to 60 percent who entered single-specialty groups/partnerships.[10] Federal efforts, such as the Health Underserved Rural Areas Program, the Rural Health Initiative, and the Community Health Centers Program have adopted the group practice format during the past decade.

The economic superiority of group practice has not as yet been convincingly demonstrated. Conceptually, economies of scale—that is, a decrease in the cost of providing medical care for a given patient

TABLE 4.11. Number of Medical Group Practices: Selected Years

Survey Year	Total Groups	Type of Specialty Group	
		Single	Multispecialty and General and Family Practice
1975	8,483[a]	4,601	3,882
1969	6,371[a]	3,169	3,202
1965	4,289[b]	2,161	2,128
1959	1,546[c]	392	1,154
1946	404[b]	36	368

Source: National Center for Health Statistics: *Health Resources Statistics, 1976–77 Edition.* USDHEW, 1979, Table 297.

[a]Three or more physicians.

[b]Three or more full-time physicians.

[c]Three physicians with two part-time physicians being counted as one full-time physician.

resulting from an increase in the amount of care provided—should result from group practice. Group practices should be able to more efficiently use personnel and equipment in "producing" medical care. Research results, however, have been mixed, and findings of economies of scale in group practice appear to be more a function of the source of data used rather than a definitive proof of the phenomenon.[48] It appears that if economies of scale do exist, benefits are maximal for small groups with three to five physicians.[49] Mixed results have also been found when comparing the productivity of solo and group practices. Accurate assessment of productivity differences as a function of group size has been stymied by the difficulty of measuring physician output as well as the inability to control for other features of group practice that may affect productivity levels, such as the use of aides and the form of payment.

Despite the lack of conclusive evidence that the formation of group practices yields economic benefits, the number of groups has grown and will continue to grow for other reasons. Health professionals currently being trained have social and professional needs that can be met more easily if they practice in a group. Group practice eases the time demands placed on the rural physician by making possible a regular schedule with guaranteed vacations, holidays, and rotating night call. But more importantly, group practice fosters the professional stimulation vital to the career development of young physicians. The daily interaction with colleagues and improved continuing medical education opportunities help to avert the provider burnout that often accompanies the long hours of solo medical practice in rural areas. This stimulation should also help to improve the quality of care delivered by the rural physician through the formal and informal review that goes on continually in a group setting.[50]

Other features of rural group practice that are of interest are their size, composition, and location. Table 4.12 presents the national distribution of medical groups by specialty and size in 1975. Although over one-half of all groups had either three or four physicians, there was a relatively wide dispersion of group size with one-fifth of all groups containing at least eight physicians. A recent, extensive nation-wide study of over 1,000 group practices by Mathematica Policy Research was unable to determine the optimal size for a group practice, as overhead costs and productivity did not vary significantly with increased group size.[51] Determination of the opti-

TABLE 4.12. Number and Percent Distribution of Medical Groups by Specialty and Size of Group: 1975

Size of Group	Total Groups		Single Specialty		General and Family Practice		Multispecialty	
	Number	Percent	Number	Percent	Number	Percent	Number	Percent
3	2,457	29.0	1,465	31.8	357	39.4	635	21.3
4	1,980	23.3	1,359	29.5	304	33.6	317	10.7
5	1,062	12.5	652	14.2	118	13.0	292	9.8
6	757	8.9	394	8.6	59	6.5	304	10.2
7	465	5.5	209	4.5	19	2.1	237	8.0
8–15	1,148	13.5	465	10.1	41	4.5	642	21.6
16–25	326	3.8	43	0.9	6	0.7	277	9.3
26–49	187	2.2	7	0.2	2	0.2	178	6.0
50–99	66	0.8	3	0.1	—	—	63	2.1
100 or more	35	0.4	4	0.1	—	—	31	1.0
Total	8,483	100.0	4,601	100.0	906	100.0	2,976	100.0

Source: National Center for Health Statistics: *Health Resources Statistics, 1976–77 Edition*. USDHEW, 1979, Table 299.

mal size and composition of a rural group practice may be only of academic interest, for many rural areas do not have a sufficient population base to support a large, or even medium-sized, multi-specialty group practice.[52] There are, of course, exceptions to this rule, with the Marshfield Clinic being a good example of a large (159 physicians) multispecialty group practice that is the major provider of medical services in a predominantly rural portion of Wisconsin.[53]

Many factors influence the location of rural group practices. On the one hand, physicians are attracted to more urbanized rural areas.[54] On the other hand, rural consumer acceptance of group practices is sensitive to travel time considerations.[55] The ability to recruit qualified physicians to join a rural group practice must be balanced against the accessibility of the group to a rural population.

In summary, the group practice concept is gaining wide acceptance. Whether group practice emerges as the solution to the problems associated with rural medical practice remains to be seen. To date, the literature suggests that the formation of a group practice does not remedy all the perceived problems of rural medical practice.[56] Group practice does, however, certainly reduce the professional isolation of the rural health professional.

The Use of Nonphysician Personnel in Rural Primary Care Practice.   Of particular importance in the development of a rural primary care practice are the decisions made by physicians concerning the number and types of nonphysician personnel who will work in the practice. The two main types of personnel that must be considered are health personnel (e.g., physician's assistants, nurse practitioners, and registered nurses) and clerical staff (e.g., receptionists and billing clerks). This section will discuss the considerations involved with the decisions to hire and use nonphysician personnel in rural primary care practice.

From a practical standpoint, the physician should have complete control of his or her style of practice. The decision to hire other personnel for a primary care practice clearly should conform to the individual practice style of the physician. In a simple, solo, fee-for-service practice, the physician may need only a receptionist/billing clerk and a registered nurse; a complex multispecialty group practice may require a variety of mid-level practitioners and a full complement of clerical help.

Reinhardt has broken down the set of tasks to be performed in a medical practice into four categories—clerical tasks, information gathering, diagnostic tasks, and therapeutic tasks.[46] He argues convincingly that tasks in each of these four categories be delegated to the lowest-skilled personnel. He finds that a significant number of physicians and other health professionals routinely perform tasks that could easily be delegated. In order to understand this paradoxical behavior, we must consider the reasons why physicians hire other professional and clerical staff and the ability of physicians to utilize these staff members efficiently once they are hired.[57]

The vast majority of clerical tasks associated with the operation of a primary care practice can be accomplished by clerical staff rather than consuming the time of the physician. The physician should, therefore, be interested in hiring clerical personnel, or equivalent outside services, to take care of functions such as appointment scheduling, billing, and bookkeeping services. The fact that most physicians adhere to this policy is reflected by the finding that 72 percent of the aggregate labor costs associated with private practices are administrative costs associated with nonmedical personnel, such as receptionists or billing clerks.[51] Nonphysician personnel make a significant contribution to physician productivity, with the optimal number of aides being almost three per physician, most of these in the nonmedical category. The major physician role in performing nonmedical tasks is managerial—acting as the leader of the practice, the individual who organizes, manages, and promotes its development.

The decision to hire other health personnel in a primary care practice is more complex than the decision to hire nonmedical personnel. The skill levels and training of other health personnel range from nurse practitioners and physician's assistants to licensed practical nurses and nurse's aides. The decision to employ other health personnel in a rural primary care practice depends on a physician's training experience, a desire to improve the operation of the practice, an attempt to increase physician income, or a desire to reduce physician workload and associated worktime.[57] Reasons for the employment of other health personnel in a rural primary care practice may not always seem completely rational. For example, many rural primary care physicians seek to hire and train registered nurses for their practices in spite of the shortage and expense of this type of health professional.[58] Moreover, the often inefficient use of registered nurses in office-based practice is suggested by the fact that many of the activities routinely performed by registered nurses (e.g., height/weight measurements, blood pressure reading, drawing of blood specimens, history taking) could be performed by staff with less training.[46]

Once the decision has been made to hire other health personnel, the physicians must develop a strategy for using these staff members in the primary care practice.[59] Physicians are forced to manage their practices and must supervise and coordinate the activities of the other health personnel in the practice. They must determine the number and types of health personnel to be hired, the timing or phase-in of personnel, and the delegation of tasks and responsibilities.

There is extensive literature concerning the use of nurse practitioners and physician's assistants in primary care practices. Although there is sufficient evidence that nurse practitioners and physician's assistants are cost effective,[60,61] provide acceptable quality of care,[62] and yield high patient satisfaction,[61] they have not been widely used in primary care practices. This conservative posture toward hiring nurse practitioners and physician's assistants can be traced to the risks the physician associates with the hiring of these personnel as well as a preference for collegial relationships. Among the risks perceived by the physician are the legal risks associated with the delegation of tasks and responsibilities to nonphysician personnel, financial concerns associated with inadequate, cumbersome reimbursement formulas, and social concerns associated with the disruption of the doctor–patient relationship and patient acceptance.[63] Faced with a growing practice, many physicians would prefer to hire another physician than to cope with these problems. Addition of another physician also increases professional stimulation and improves the ability of the practice to provide systematic coverage on a continuous basis.

Golladay et al. describe the physician as a conservative economic agent.[64] This frequently results in a sizable gap between what a physician could delegate to nonphysicians, and what in fact the physician does delegate. From the economist's viewpoint this causes an inefficient use of physician and nonphysician time in office-based primary care practice. The physician is clearly motivated by considerations that go beyond simple economic efficiency and it is unlikely that this will change in the near future.

The Financial Viability of Rural Primary Care.   One of the major goals of a new rural primary care practice is to attain financial self-sufficiency. In order to accomplish that goal, a short-term and a long-term strategy must be developed.

The first year of operation of a rural primary care practice is an exciting yet often unstable period. It is a time of erratic growth—a period during which the practice and the community start to reach a balance with one another. It is not unusual during the first year of operation for rural primary care practices to collect as little as one-half to one-third of their gross charges, to see as few as 10 to 12 patients per day per physician, and to have net receipts covering only half of the total expenses associated with the practice.[65] The rural primary care practice often needs help to sustain itself during this initial stage.

A sizable proportion of total costs associated with a primary care practice is fixed.[58] This is particularly the case at the outset of a practice when the fixed costs of space, equipment, and personnel are extremely high compared to the variable costs associated with running the practice. This is the time when strong community involvement with the planning process can pay off. New rural primary care practices need external support to offset their high starting costs. This support can come in the form of rent-free space or inexpensive equipment and supplies. This support can also indicate community interest in the survival of the practice and help to alter the health care utilization patterns of local residents over time.

As practices mature, emphasis can be placed on monitoring and controlling key fiscal parameters. These parameters include gross charges, net receipts, total expenses, and volume of patient encounters. Our own previous research on the growth and development of rural primary care practices suggests that they grow slowly but steadily over time.[65,66] Table 4.13 summarizes the results of those studies and indicates that, after two years of growth, rural primary care practices can expect approximately 1,000 patients per quarter per provider full-time equivalent (FTE). After two years, gross charges were in the neighborhood of $20,000 per quarter per FTE, and the collection rate was almost 85 percent. The major differences observed in the different settings we studied were in the values of practice expense ratios, more commonly referred to as overhead, which ranged from approximately .55 to .75 after two years. The differences in expense ratios were also reflected in the values of practice self-sufficiency at

TABLE 4.13. The Growth of Rural Primary Care Practices

	Practice Age				
	$\frac{1}{2}$ Year	1 Year	1½ Years	2 Years	2½ Years
Gross charges per FTE					
National Health Service Corps (NHSC)[a]	11,555	16,498	17,991	18,364	—
Rural Practice Project (RPP)[b]	15,352	19,016	18,601	21,878	22,402
Practice collection ratio					
NHSC	.62	.67	.73	.84	—
RPP	.73	.85	.88	.84	.92
Number patient encounters per FTE					
NHSC	642	819	909	978	—
RPP	845	1,015	951	1,053	967
Practice expense ratio					
NHSC	.75	.68	.55	.56	—
RPP	1.04	1.09	.80	.73	.66
Practice self-sufficiency ratio					
NHSC	.45	.63	.75	.87	—
RPP	.45	.53	.62	.64	.74

Definitions:

Practice collection ratio = $\dfrac{\text{net receipts}}{\text{gross charges}}$

Practice expense ratio = $\dfrac{\text{total expenses}}{\text{gross charges}}$

Practice self-sufficiency ratio = $\dfrac{\text{net receipts}}{\text{total expenses} + \text{provider salaries}}$

[a] Refers to a study of nine National Health Service Corps sites. See Rosenblatt R, Moscovice I: The growth and evolution of rural primary care practice—The NHSC experience in the Northwest. *Medical Care* 16:819–827, 1978.

[b] Refers to a study of nine Robert Wood Johnson Foundation Rural Practice Projects. See Moscovice I, Rosenblatt R: Rural health care delivery amidst federal retrenchment: Lessons from the Robert Wood Johnson Foundation's Rural Practice Project. *Am J Pub Health*, forthcoming.

two years, which ranged from .64 for sites with high overhead to .87 for sites with fewer administrative costs.

Table 4.13 indicates that there is steady improvement in the financial viability of rural primary care practices in their early years of operation. With similar continued growth, the majority of rural practices that were studied would attain financial self-sufficiency in three to five years. It is important to note that these data reflect the growth patterns of rural primary care practices that were established in underserved areas and received external support from their first day of operation. If anything, one would expect primary care practices established in better served, more densely populated rural areas to attain financial equilibrium more easily.

Environmental characteristics not readily controlled by the physician also affect rural practices. The primary environmental factor that influences the financial success or failure of rural primary care practice is the size and structure of the service area population. It has been shown that a minimum population size of 4,000 is necessary to support a two-person rural physician practice.[65,67] A rural primary care practice with a service area population of 4,000 and an average of three to four visits per year per person, with a charge of $15 per office visit and a collection rate of 85 percent, should be able to generate the gross income of $150,000 to $170,000 necessary for support of the practice.[32] Below this threshold a rural primary care practice cannot be expected to generate the income necessary to cover overhead expenses and provider salaries and will, therefore, require continued external support for sustenance.

The structure of the service area population is also of importance. Kane et al. suggest that rural areas with the fewest resources will have the most difficulty in recruiting and retaining physicians.[5] These areas will have a difficult time not only in attracting health professionals but also in supporting financially viable practices. From a practical perspective, a rural primary care practice needs a broad patient population base comprised of upper-, middle-, and lower-income groups. If the upper- and middle-income groups seek health care in larger cities outside the local service area, the practice will not survive.

Another significant environmental factor that affects the financial viability of rural primary care practice is the availability of other health resources, such as hospitals, nursing homes, and other social service facilities. The rural physician uses the local hospital and nursing home as a second "office." This second office can be quite profitable because it is free of overhead expense for the rural physician and can often provide the extra income necessary for sustaining the practice. Our earlier research found that the absence of a local hospital limited the growth capabilities of a rural primary care practice and that the supply of hospital beds readily available to the physician was positively related to the economic performance of the primary care practitioner.[65,66] Wallack and Kretz find that self-sufficient rural practices generate more than one-third of their total revenues from hospitals.[37] Practices that did not have this source of income had difficulty achieving financial solvency. Rural primary care practices often depend on the hospital's "free workshop" for their economic viability.

For the most part, the environmental characteristics described above can be considered fixed. The physician generally finds himself in a position of being responsive to these factors rather than being able to control them. The second set of factors that affects the financial viability of rural primary care is controlled by the physician. These factors are related to the way the practice is organized, the resources it utilizes, and the services it provides. A major pitfall is the development of excess capacity in facilities, equipment, and personnel in the initial period of operation of a rural primary care practice. Resources need to be phased in as a practice matures. Excessive building costs should be avoided if possible during the initial, unstable period of practice growth. Office staff can be incrementally added as required by the practice, and on-site laboratory and x-ray facilities are profitable for the primary care practice only once a sufficient patient load is established.

It has been shown that the scope of services provided in a rural primary care practice influences the fiscal viability of the practice. Practices that provide significant amounts of preventive care and outreach services have difficulty achieving economic self-sufficiency.[52] The reimbursement system discriminates against the provision of these basic primary care services. Practices that provide hospital-based services are able to attain self-sufficiency with less difficulty than practices that do not provide these services.

Practice organizational structure should also be expected to influence the economic characteristics of a primary care practice; however, studies to date have had mixed results concerning the impact of some of the major organizational variables on financial viability. In an earlier section we discussed the lack of clear-cut data documenting the existence of economies of scale in group practice. From a purely financial perspective, the superiority of group practice over solo practice has not been established. Another key organizational variable believed to improve financial viability is the degree of administrative expertise of the professional staff of the primary care practice. Many physicians lack these skills, which are rarely addressed during training. It is difficult to quantify the contributions of management expertise to the economic growth of rural primary care practice, and the cost effectiveness of hiring a professional administrator capable of providing management leadership depends on many factors, including the number of physicians in the practice.[66]

A final organizational variable that affects economic viability is the reward system, or salary structure, associated with the practice. Rural providers need an incentive to overcome the obstacles encountered in building a primary care practice. For some providers, these incentives are financial, and fixed salaries may prove to be an insufficient stimulus. Hence, it has been suggested that one reasonable approach to salary structure, particularly in group practices, is to provide a base-line pay level with additional monetary incentives based on productivity levels.[36]

During the past decade an increasing number of rural areas have attracted primary care physicians. There are, and will continue to be, a set of rural areas that cannot sustain the development of private primary care physician practices. Areas with populations fewer than 4,000, with no hospital facilities, and located more than 15 to 20 miles from a larger city fall in this category. These communities will require external support if their residents are to have adequate access to primary care services. The current focus on cost containment will undoubtedly exacerbate the health care delivery problems of these areas if the result is a limitation on the amount, length, and type of external support provided to these communities.

Alternatives to the Rural Entrepreneurial Model.   It is impossible to define the "typical" rural community. Rural communities are diverse, and there are a variety of health care delivery models that can meet the primary care needs of these communities. The previous sections described significant issues involved with the development of rural primary care practices by the private sector. This section will discuss four alternatives to the traditional rural physician model:

1. Hospital-based primary care
2. Health maintenance organizations
3. Nonphysician personnel in a remote clinic
4. Public and private foundation efforts

Hospital-Based Primary Care.   As access to primary care became a central health policy issue in the 1970s, various innovative approaches were developed to meet the primary care needs of underserved populations. One of these approaches was the concept of hospital-based primary care. The community hospital was identified as a logical base for the provision of primary health care services.[68] Traditionally, large urban hospitals maintain sizable outpatient departments and emergency rooms that provide a wide array of ambulatory care services. The use of these services increased more than fourfold during the period 1965–76.[69] This experience led to expansion of the concept of hospital-based primary care, going beyond the traditional hospital outpatient department. Reorganization of an existing outpatient department or the development of medical group practices affiliated with the hospital were two new organizational frameworks proposed for the delivery of hospital-based primary care.

The rationale for delivering hospital-based primary care is not as clear cut in rural areas. Traditionally, the rural hospital has not played as large a role in the delivery of ambulatory care. Few rural hospitals have formally organized outpatient departments, and many have inadequate, poorly staffed emergency rooms. Nonetheless, the rural hospital has been forced to look for ways to improve access to primary care for its service area population.[70] Hospital-based primary care could become a reality for those rural hospitals willing to accept the challenge of expanding their mission and providing needed services for the community. In this sense, though, it must be viewed as a "loss leader." There are no guarantees of increased hospital admissions or greater use of hospital ancillary services directly attributable to the provision of hospital-based primary care.

Madison and Bernstein have identified three major forms for hospital-based primary care in rural areas.[71] The first is the hospital-based, physician-sponsored program like the Marshfield Clinic in Wisconsin or the Geisinger Clinic in Pennsylvania. In these examples, the hospital incorporates a sizable multispecialty group practice in or adjacent to its inpatient facility, with the hospital and group being linked by an affiliation-type agreement concerning the use of facilities, equipment, support services, and so forth. The second is the hospital-based, hospital-sponsored program (e.g., Indian Health Service clinics in the Southwest and Alaska), which builds on an existing capability of the hospital to deliver primary care. This framework is not as common as the first due to the lack of existing organizational frameworks for the delivery of primary care in most rural hospitals. The third is the primary care satellite facility sponsored by the hospital to improve access to health care for medically underserved, often isolated populations. Examples include the satellite facilities sponsored by Rural Health Associates of Maine and the Bolivar Clinic sponsored by Mercy Hospital in Pennsylvania.

Rural hospital-based primary care programs must overcome a formidable group of obstacles. These include physician recruitment and retention problems inherent to rural areas, local physician opposition, the unstable financial position of many rural hospitals, lack of hospital administrative knowledge and experience regarding primary care, and hospital/primary care group turf battles relating to the degree of group autonomy.[71,72] In addition, accurate data are virtually nonexistent concerning the costs involved with the delivery of hospital-based primary care and the impact of these programs on the financial position of the rural hospital.[69] The Robert Wood Johnson Foundation is currently sponsoring an evaluation of its Medical Staff Sponsored Primary Care Group Practice Program that will help to quantify the impact of hospital-based primary care from an institutional and community perspective.[72]

One-fifth of all hospitals in the United States anticipate establishing primary care group practices in the near future.[73] The rural hospital will undoubtedly play a larger role in the delivery of primary care in the 1980s.[74] The primary benefit that the hospital can achieve from this change is its enhanced role as a significant community resource—as an integral part of the health care system. The community can benefit from improved access to primary care as well as from the effective integration of ambulatory and inpatient services it receives.

Health Maintenance Organizations.   During the 1970s, the federal government made strong efforts to foster the development of health maintenance organizations. Enrollment in HMOs more than doubled during the 1970s. An HMO can be defined as "an organization that accepts the contractual responsibility for making available and providing to all enrollees a specified range of medical care services (usually at least ambulatory and inpatient services) at an identified location(s) in return for their prepaid capitation payments."[75]

There are two main organizational structures for HMOs. The most common is the prepaid group practice in which physicians are usually on salary and share space, equipment, and/or personnel. The second is the Independent Practice Association (IPA), or foundation for medical care, under which enrollees make capitation payments and receive health care services from private physicians who are members of the IPA. IPA physicians have their own fee-for-service practice and are paid according to a predetermined fee schedule for their IPA patients.

Conceptually, HMOs have been viewed as organizations that will improve the access and continuity of health services by identifying a regular source of care for all enrollees, and that will save money by altering the financial incentives for health providers. In a recent review, Luft suggests there is good evidence that HMO enrollees incur lower total health care costs than their non-HMO counterparts primarily due to one-third fewer hospital days per 1,000 population; however, the differences observed have been dependent on the particular plan studied and range anywhere from 10–40 percent.[49] In addition, the impact of consumer self-selection to HMOs has not been adequately addressed, making it difficult to accurately assess the impact of the HMO delivery form on health care costs. It is also not clear that HMOs have been successful in improving access. Although out-of-plan usage and voluntary disenrollment from HMO plans has been quite low, HMO enrollees are less satisfied with their geographic access to medical care and with appointment waiting time.

Despite the fact that previous attempts at the development of capitated health plans had been largely unsuccessful in rural areas, the passage of the HMO Act of 1973 (PL 93–222) offered new hope for rural HMOs. This act required that employees of businesses with 25 or more staff members be offered, whenever feasible, an HMO plan as a health insurance option. Moreover, funds were made available for HMO feasibility surveys (up to $50,000 for each project), planning for expansion of existing HMOs and initial development costs of new HMOs (up to $125,000 for expansion projects, up to $1 million for initial development projects), and loans for initial operational losses and loan guarantees for initial operations of HMOs in medically underserved areas (up to $1 million annually for each project). For the period 1975–80, there have been 615 feasibility and planning and development grants totaling $127.8 million, 91 loans for HMO operations totaling $168.5 million, and five loan guarantees to HMOs in medically underserved areas totaling $7.8 million.[76]

The 1973 HMO Act set aside 20 percent of all funds for the planning, development, and operation of rural HMOs and gave priority to applications from HMOs that would be developed in medically underserved areas. Despite these good intentions, it became quickly apparent that there were major obstacles to the development of rural HMOs. Rural HMOs are a riskier proposition than their urban counterparts. Many of the same problems facing the private physician also face the developers of the rural health maintenance organization. Rural areas have an inadequate supply of physicians, troubled hospitals, a limited economic base, and sparsely settled populations that are often resistant to attempts to change the status quo.[77] Furthermore, some of the federal HMO requirements, such as the provision of a comprehensive benefit package including mental health and drug and alcohol abuse treatment and a payment mechanism fixed on a community rating basis, are impractical for rural areas.

Despite the lack of overall success of the federal HMO effort in rural areas, there are examples of successful rural HMOs. Among these are

1. North Quabbin Health Plan (NQHP), serving a nine-town area with 23,000 residents in northern Massachusetts.[78] NQHP was

started in 1973 and is a prepaid health plan that established a hospital-based primary care center. Physicians in the plan can work on salary or on a fee-for-service basis, and subscriber eligibility and premiums vary with subscriber income.

2. Greater Marshfield Community Health Plan (GMCHP), serving a 30-township area of over 3,000 square miles in central Wisconsin.[79] This plan was established in 1971 and has expanded dramatically, having enrolled 44,000 of the 112,000 residents of the area.[53] The plan is community rated with a two-step premium structure for single persons and families. It was established as a collaborative venture of the Marshfield Clinic, St. Joseph's Hospital (a 434-bed facility), and Wisconsin Blue Cross/Blue Shield. The plan capitalized on the strong reputation of the Marshfield Clinic, a successful multispecialty group practice that has served the same area for over 50 years.

3. Valley Health Plan, serving the university community and residents of the semirural area surrounding Amherst, Massachusetts, since 1976.[80] This plan was based on a unique liaison between a private group practice and a public university student health program and emphasized using the marginal capacity of existing health resources in the community to their fullest extent. The plan had a market penetration of over 40 percent of eligible enrollees at the university and small businesses in the area and broke even financially after only one year of operation.

Other groups still maintain strong interest in developing rural HMOs. These include the continued efforts of Rural Health Associates in Maine to develop a prepaid health plan that would serve up to 50 percent of the 30,000 members of its service area population in central Maine and attempts to develop a prepaid health plan—the Great Valley Health Plan (GVHP)—to provide health care to low-income rural and migrant families in six rural counties in the San Joaquin Valley in California.[81] The GVHP service area has approximately 142,000 Medi-Cal recipients who would be eligible for the plan. They would receive care in three health centers and four satellite offices that are currently part of a consortium of clinics that are members of a private nonprofit corporation, the California Rural Health Federation.

In reviewing the experience of the few successful existing rural HMOs and those currently in the planning stage, a set of factors emerge that appear to be related to a successful venture. First, there must be an adequate supply of primary care providers in a rural area willing to provide the majority of services required.[82] Second, although it is impossible to provide all services locally, improving the use of any underutilized capacity (e.g., hospital inpatient facilities, emergency room, and nursing service) in the service area is desirable.[78] Third, a broad base of community and industry support is necessary from a political and actuarial standpoint.[83] Fourth, an appropriate and flexible organizational structure must be developed for the rural HMO. For example, rural HMOs could be set up by expanding already existing "parent" HMOs located in urban areas or through creation of innovative arrangements involving the use of IPAs. Fifth, the burden of capital investment should be minimized in the initial stages of growth of a rural HMO.[80] Finally, realistic forecasts of subscriber enrollment accompanied by effective marketing techniques are essential to planning and implementation efforts.

As we have shown, the development of an HMO may not be a practical solution to meet the primary care needs of most rural areas. Nonetheless, there are examples of successful rural HMOs that show that in carefully selected settings the HMO may be a feasible alternative. Rural leaders should give consideration to the HMO approach, particularly given the current emphasis on market-oriented solutions to the escalating costs of health care delivery.

Nonphysician Personnel in a Remote Area Clinic.   At present, shortages of health care manpower still exist in many isolated small towns, particularly those lacking hospital facilities or the economic base to support a group of physicians. The problem of gaining access to the traditional health care delivery system is particularly acute for the more remote rural communities.

One potential solution is the use of nurse practitioners and physician's assistants for the delivery of primary health care services. A major impetus for the development of these new types of health care personnel was the shortage of primary care physicians in rural areas and inner cities. Midlevel practitioner programs have proliferated in the past few years, stimulated by private and federal grants (Table 4.14). Most of these practitioners have been absorbed into

TABLE 4.14. Present and Projected Supply of Physician Assistants and Nurse Practitioners: 1975, 1980, and 1990

	1975	1980	Basic	1990 Low	1990 High
Total midlevel practitioners	7,640	18,840	41,550	29,040	57,590
Total physician assistants (PAs)	2,540	7,410	18,520	13,200	27,700
Physician assistants	2,100	6,550	16,640	11,790	26,440
MEDEX	440	860	1,880	1,410	2,860
Total nurse practitioners (NPs)	5,100	11,430	23,030	15,840	29,890
NP certificate	3,800	8,270	15,680	11,140	20,210
NP masters	1,300	3,160	6,350	4,700	8,680

Source: On the Status of Health Professions Personnel in the United States, A Report to the President and Congress, Health Resources Administration, USDHHS, August 1978, Table 10.

larger institutional settings or incorporated into the existing practices of rural and urban physicians.

Midlevel practitioners, particularly those in solo practices in isolated areas, confront many of the same problems that led to the declining number of solo general practitioners. These obstacles include professional isolation, a lack of opportunity for professional growth, legal barriers to the establishment of midlevel practices, problems of community acceptance, and marginal financial viability.

Professional isolation is perhaps the key factor that undermines solo physician practice and is one of the most difficult barriers for the solo midlevel provider to overcome. The remote solo practitioner has major difficulties in overcoming professional isolation. Coverage arrangements are cumbersome, requiring formal short-term replacement agreements with distant practitioners. Consultation requires a phone call or patient referral. The ongoing stimulation of informal professional interrelationships is not readily available.

An important component of an isolated solo midlevel practice is the development of strong linkages with surrounding health care providers and facilities. If nearby physicians view the midlevel provider as an economic competitor or a threat to the provision of high quality care, they will not accept the practitioner as a primary care provider. If they view the midlevel provider as a complement to their roles as primary care providers, then cooperation, encouragement, backup, and consultation and referral arrangements should result.

Rural practice is demanding. The solo physician grew weary of 24-hour on-call responsibility, often augmented by hospital responsibilities. Kane has pointed out that the value of midlevel providers in remote settings is directly related to the degree to which they can work without direct physician supervision.[62] However, the midlevel provider will require interprofessional collaboration and cooperation from physicians to overcome the overwhelming sense of responsibility attendant upon being the solo health provider in an isolated community. Rural health care delivery is fragile at best and can exist only by forging effective links between all components of the health care system.

Professional growth is one area in which midlevel practitioners have a theoretical advantage over their solo physician counterparts. Nurse practitioners and physician's assistants may find an isolated, relatively independent primary care practice a challenging setting for the practice of their profession. Rather than a professional backwater, the remote practice is an opportunity to grapple with difficult clinical problems and attempt to work through them independently. If appropriately linked with ready consultation, an accessible continuing education program, and periodic peer relationships, a remote area assignment could prove to be professionally attractive.

One barrier to the use of solo midlevel practitioners in remote practices has been legal restrictions placed on the practice of medicine by nonphysicians. Leitch and Mitchell have shown that laws and regulations are changing rapidly but inconsistently in the effort to facilitate the expansion of nursing roles.[84] By 1977, over 30 states had revised their nurse practice acts to facilitate role expansion. Only half of the remaining states explicitly prohibit a nurse from diagnosing and treating a medical condition. Nonetheless, the number of constraints on the scope of practice (ability to prescribe medications, order laboratory tests, etc.) of a nurse practitioner varies considerably from state to state.

Kissam found that at least 37 states had enacted physician's assistant (PA) statutes by the summer of 1975.[85] Many of these statutes give medical licensing boards the authority to oversee the practices of physician's assistants. In terms of remote practices, these boards can define acceptable modes of supervision that enable physician's assistants to practice under the guidance of a physician who is not on the premises.

A range of formal professional relationships exists in isolated practices. In some cases, the remote practitioner is under the direct supervision of a distant physician; in other cases, the practitioner is theoretically independent. The important point is that the actual operating relationship often depends on the personalities of the individuals involved—and the demographics of the situation—rather than the formal legal relationships in force. Legal restrictions, on the other hand, inhibit the entry of midlevel providers into solo, remote practice.

Critical to the success of a remote midlevel practice are community acceptance and support. Populations in isolated rural communities have become accustomed to satisfying their health care needs by traveling to remote trade centers, using nontraditional sources of care, such as chiropractors and naturopaths, or managing without direct access to primary care services. Conservative rural communities will not readily disrupt their current health care seeking behavior to uncritically embrace the solo, midlevel provider.

Midlevel providers have lower salary expectations than physicians, and they can attain financial stability with fewer patients. Remote clinics, however, have been characterized by small operating budgets, few auxiliary staff, low fee levels, poor collection rates, and limited productivity, which tend to undermine economic success.[86] Schweitzer and Record have suggested that a major impediment to the growth of such clinics is the refusal of most third-party payers to reimburse directly for services.[87] Even recent legislation (PL 95–210, Rural Health Clinics Services Act) aimed at expanding the availability of medical and nursing care in physician-underserved areas has done little to improve reimbursement to remote clinics not under the direct control of physicians. Under this bill, the clinic, and not the midlevel provider, is reimbursed by Medicare and Medicaid for services furnished by the midlevel provider. Moreover, many services (e.g., nursing home calls, counseling activities, diet control, health education, and chronic illness maintenance) that can be provided by nurse practitioners are reimbursed at low levels or not at all.

Our previous research on the economic viability of remote midlevel practices established by the National Health Service Corps in the Pacific Northwest indicated that low productivity (approximately 10 to 12 patients per working day) and high overhead reduced the chances of economic self-sufficiency of these practices.[88] In addition, we found that a minimum population size of 1,500 was required for isolated midlevel practices to be able to attain financial self-sufficiency without continuing external subsidy.

An interesting example of an established system of midlevel practitioner clinics is the 17 remote midlevel clinics built in North Carolina with the support of the State Office of Rural Health Services.[89] These clinics provide primary care services on a continuing basis to over 50,000 rural residents in North Carolina and are an excellent example of a primary care delivery program effectively utilizing midlevel practitioners.

One study of the use of a nurse practitioner in a remote rural community points out the deleterious impact of reimbursement practices on the viability of the nonphysician practice in rural areas.[90] The study documents the replacement of a solo, National Health

Service Corps (NHSC) physician in a small rural community in eastern Oregon by a nurse practitioner. Within two years the nurse practitioner increased practice productivity and charges by more than 40 percent, yet the practitioner left the community one year later. The major factors underlying this turn of events were the nurse practitioner's ineligibility for Medicare reimbursement and an inability to sign prescriptions under the state's pharmacy statutes. Thus despite excellent community acceptance, the midlevel practice was unable to achieve financial and professional stability.

To summarize, the use of nurse practitioners or physician's assistants can be a feasible way to provide primary care services to geographically isolated populations. Physicians must provide strong support to help the isolated midlevel practice overcome professional and legal obstacles if this approach is to work. Even with this support, external subsidies may be necessary if primary health care services are to be made readily accessible to remote populations.

Public and Private Foundation Efforts.   During the past 20 years there have been many public efforts aimed at improving the delivery of primary care in rural areas. Our summary here of these recent efforts adds to our earlier discussions of these programs in Chapter 2.

In 1976, Lee et al. identified 24 federal departments and agencies that were responsible for programs attempting to improve health care delivery in rural areas.[3] These programs worked primarily in two ways: by funding the training of primary care providers and by establishing primary health care delivery programs. The major effort in the area of training was designed to encourage the preparation of a new generation of family physicians and the creation of new kinds of midlevel practitioners. Public Law 94–484, passed in 1976, required that at least 50 percent of first-year residency training slots be in primary care specialties if medical schools wished to receive capitation funds and other federal training support. The two largest funding categories for health professions special project authorizations for fiscal years 1978–80 were family medicine residencies at $140 million and Physician Assistant, Expanded Function Dental Auxiliaries, and Team Approaches at $90 million.[91]

In addition to bolstering the support for the training of primary care providers, the federal government also expanded the scope and influence of a number of service delivery programs.[92] The

NHSC—the centerpiece of this effort—was created by the Emergency Health Personnel Act (PL 91–623) of 1970 to improve rural health care by developing self-sufficient primary care practices in underserved areas. NHSC-sponsored practices were initially expected to become financially independent after two to four years of federal support. The NHSC differed from previous federal efforts in that it directly placed health providers in rural areas rather than providing funds for the development of health care delivery programs.

PL 94–484 dramatically increased the size and changed the focus of the NHSC program (see Table 4.15). The NHSC was transformed from an agency developing freestanding rural primary care practices to the health manpower staffing source for all federal rural health projects. The NHSC became a central component in the federal strategy for integrating the fragmented federal rural health efforts. The addition of a large scholarship program insured a steady stream of recent medical graduates for federal projects.

This new federal strategy developed in conjunction with the Rural Health Initiative (RHI), an administrative effort of the Bureau of Community Health Services (BCHS) to develop local capacity to build and maintain rural health systems by integrating a variety of BCHS categorical programs that affected rural health care.[23] Among the categorical programs that were tapped in the effort to combine personnel, facilities, and support services at the local level were the Community Health Centers Program, National Health Service Corps, Migrant Health Program, and Appalachian Health Program.

The two major programs that provided the bulk of the funding and manpower for the RHI were the NHSC and the Community Health Centers (CHC) programs. CHCs were an outgrowth of the Neighborhood Health Center Program originally administered by the now defunct Office of Economic Opportunity and are currently authorized under Section 330 of the Public Health Service Act.[5] The NHSC, as described earlier, was used as the personnel source for RHI projects. The CHC program was used to provide grant support for ambulatory care projects in medically underserved areas. CHC grants were used for the planning, development, and operation of ambulatory care clinics and required that eligible projects provide a comprehensive range of services, including primary medical care, dental care, prescription drugs, mental health services, outreach ser-

TABLE 4.15. Growth of the NHSC Program

Item						Year				
	1971	1972	1973	1974	1975	1976	1976[a]	1977	1978	1979
NHSC field appropriations ($ million)	3	12.6	11	13	15	20	9	25	41	65
NHSC scholarship appropriations ($ million)	—	—	—	3	23	23	23	40	60	75
Total federal assignees in field	—	34	150	338	470	611	—	724	1,289	1,725
Number of new scholarship recipients	—	—	—	1,870	871	885	—	2,089	3,346	2,379

Source: Rosenblatt R, Moscovice I: The National Health Service Corps: Rapid growth and uncertain future. *Milbank Memorial Fund Quarterly* 58:283–309, 1980, Table 1.

[a]Transitional quarter.

vices, nutrition programs, transportation services, environmental health services, home health services, and child development programs.[16]

The support for Community Health Centers nearly tripled (from $110 million to $320 million) in the period 1973–80, and in recent years the program has increasingly focused on rural areas. Two-thirds (575 of 872) of CHCs in 1980 were in nonmetropolitan communities.[93] CHCs serve predominantly low-income populations that have complex health problems, language difficulties, and other sociocultural barriers hindering access to health care. Initial studies have indicated that these efforts have had a positive impact on health status while providing services in a cost-effective fashion.[94]

Several of the more narrow categorical programs have not been as readily integrated into the Rural Health Initiative program. One example is the Migrant Health Center program (MHC). The Migrant Health Act (PL 87–692), passed in 1962, provided a small amount of funds for state and county health departments to work on communicable disease control among the migrant population. The enactment of PL 91–209 in 1970 changed the program focus significantly, authorizing the development of community-based comprehensive primary care programs for migrants.[95] The act also extended eligibility to seasonal farmworkers and their families, thereby increasing the population served by Migrant Health Centers from 102,000 in 1970 to over 550,000 by 1978.[96]

Currently, centers that are eligible for funding by the Migrant Health Center program must be located in federally designated high impact areas that contain at least 4,000 migrants and/or seasonal farmworkers and their families for at least two months of the year. The funding for the Migrant Health Center program has gradually increased during recent years and was $39.7 million for fiscal year 1980.[93] Supporters of the Migrant Health Center program have opposed the diversion of funds from the Migrant Health Center program to RHI, even though most migrants are in rural areas.[95]

Table 4.16 shows the growth of selected BCHS categorical programs and RHI projects over the period 1975–80. Despite scattered opposition, the RHI effort has expanded dramatically in recent years and has been considered by many to be a conceptually creative approach to the management of BCHS resources. RHI may not, however, have the long-range stability necessary to build rural health

TABLE 4.16. Growth of BCHS Programs, 1975–80

Program	1975		1977		1979		1980	
	Number of Projects	Funding Level ($ million)	Number of Projects	Funding Level ($ million)	Number of Projects	Funding Level ($ million)	Number of Projects	Funding Level ($ million)
Rural health initiative	47	7.2	262	23.6	397	43.1	526	63.7
Community health centers	204	196.6	455	215.1	632	253.0	872	320.0
Health underserved rural areas	9	3.3	88	15.0	104	16.5	66	14.0
Migrant health	105	23.8	105	30.0	112	34.5	122	39.7

Source: Bureau of Community Health Services, DHHS, 1981.

systems because it lacks a statutory funding base. The future of both the RHI and the traditional categorical programs is uncertain, and it is highly likely that they will be radically altered by the current "cut, cap, and block grant" approach of federal policy makers. As these programs are transferred to state control, and their funding levels severely curtailed, it is impossible to predict what shape they will take in the coming decade.

In addition to federal efforts, an increasing number of states are becoming directly involved with attempts to improve rural health care. Colorado, California, Wyoming, Nevada, and New Mexico have developed Offices of Rural Health based on the successful model established in North Carolina. These agencies have become involved with the development of programs to strengthen the recruitment and retention of physicians, nurses, and other health personnel in rural areas, and they are also attempting to coordinate federal efforts within their borders. A good example of state-federal cooperation is the development of Area Health Education Centers, which decentralize health professional educational training opportunities, link rural health providers and facilities with large urban health resource centers, and work with the National Health Service Corps to place physicians in underserved areas.[26]

State and local health departments have also substantially increased their roles in the direct provision of medical services, including primary care. The traditional role of public health departments has included communicable disease control, environmental sanitation, maternal and child health services, health education, vital statistics, and laboratory services.[97] Several states (e.g., North Carolina, Georgia, and Tennessee) have recently expanded the role of health departments to include the provision of primary care services in rural areas.[98] In Tennessee, the Department of Public Health established a network of rural primary care centers staffed primarily by nurse practitioners.[29] In North Carolina, 20 of the 81 local health departments have received funds from the State Health Services Division to implement a variety of rural primary care programs designed to meet the health care needs of individual communities.[98,99]

Private foundations have also supported the development of alternative delivery systems in rural areas. Two major national efforts have been sponsored by the Sears Roebuck Foundation and the Robert Wood Johnson Foundation. From 1957–70, the Sears

Roebuck Foundation developed and equipped modern practice facilities in rural areas to help improve the recruitment and retention of physicians. Twenty percent of the 163 rural areas that built clinics were not able to attract physicians to their towns, and turnover was high among those physicians who were recruited.[28] The construction of a modern facility in itself was an inadequate solution to the problem of health care delivery in rural areas.

In 1975, the Robert Wood Johnson Foundation initiated the Rural Practice Project (RPP), which provided grants to 13 physician and health administrator teams to develop multidisciplinary practices in rural communities spread across the United States. The RPP emphasized the importance of creating leadership teams as the core of a successful, community-responsive rural practice. RPP sites have grown slowly but steadily during their first few years. Economic self-sufficiency should be attained by the majority of sites by the end of several years of operation.[66] One deterrent to financial equilibrium has been the high overhead of RPP sites due to the costs of maintaining a full-time administrator at each site.

In summary, there have been many public and private attempts to improve the delivery of rural primary care. These programs have made primary care available to many rural citizens, but significant gaps remain.[94] Public and private efforts to improve rural health care would benefit from increased coordination. This is particularly true in an era when federal support for rural health is waning. The promising rural health projects started in the 1970s can be continued only if local communities and state and local government begin to play a more central role.

CONCLUSIONS

Primary care services are the basic foundation of the rural health system. The primary care practice is the entry point to the health care system for most rural dwellers. Primary care services should be accessible to the population residing in rural areas. Accessibility to primary care should not be sacrificed simply because it may cost more to provide health care services in rural areas.

Rural communities must be willing to share with health providers the risk involved in the development of primary care programs. Communities must use their strengths and capabilities to help assure the viability of rural primary care. They must be willing to plan, design, implement, maintain, and use their primary care programs.

Rural providers must be patient and flexible in their approach to program development. They must be able to weather the crises that arise during the initial stages of program operation. Rural primary care programs should utilize generalists capable of providing a broad range of services and must be integrated within a rural health system that has developed the necessary linkages with other clinical, professional, and management services.

We have learned a great deal from the rural health programs of the 1970s. The following list summarizes some of those lessons:

1. Primary care services can be provided to rural communities. Access to primary care services in rural areas has improved steadily over time.
2. Despite good intentions, programs driven by external forces can have a deleterious effect on the natural development of rural health care systems. Local community involvement and support are necessary for the continued life of a rural primary care program. Decentralization of responsibility for program management and operation should take place as early as possible.
3. New rural primary care practices grow slowly but steadily. Patience is required to survive the three- to five-year maturation process that usually leads to practice stability. Some rural communities will always require external support for the maintenance of health care services.
4. It is difficult to alter the basic way medical services are provided without accompanying changes in reimbursement policies. There is an urgent need to improve financing for primary care services.
5. The maldistribution of health resources is not easily overcome. Rural areas depend on the training of sufficient generalists to assure an adequate supply of health manpower.
6. Approaches that attack one particular aspect of the rural primary care problem, such as the lack of appropriate personnel or facilities, often provide fragmented short-term "solutions" to long-term problems. The temptation to deal with immediate concerns

must be carefully balanced against the need for thoughtful long-range planning.

There are many alternative ways to provide primary care in a rural area. The selection of the best approach is a delicate process that must involve the affected community.

REFERENCES

1. Stumbo WG: Rural health centers and the development of progressive patient care. *Clinical Medicine* 84:10–13, 1977.
2. Scheffler R, Weisfeld N, Ruby G, et al: A manpower policy for primary health care. *New England Journal of Medicine* 298:1058–1062, 1978.
3. Lee P, LeRoy L, Stalcup J, Beck J: *Primary Care in a Specialized World.* Cambridge, Mass, Ballinger, 1976.
4. Bureau of Community Health Services: *Building a Rural Health System.* Rockville, Md, USDHEW, Health Services Administration, 1976.
5. Kane R, Dean M, Solomon M: An evaluation of rural health care research. *Evaluation Quarterly* 3:139–189, 1979.
6. Rosenblatt R: Planning ensures local and referral care for remote rural area. *Hospitals* 53:83–88, 1979.
7. Ferreti W: The realities of rural primary care. *Journal of Ambulatory Care Management* 2:29–38, 1979.
8. Hobbs D: Rural development: Intentions and consequences. *Rural Sociology* 45:7–25, 1980.
9. Scheffler R, Yoder S, Weisfeld N, et al: Physicians and new health practitioners: Issues for the 1980's. *Inquiry* 16:195–229, 1979.
10. Geyman J: Family practice in evolution—Progress, problems, and projections. *New England Journal of Medicine* 298:593–601, 1978.
11. Coleman S: *Physician Distribution and Rural Access to Medical Services.* Santa Monica, Calif, Rand Corporation, 1976.
12. Madison D: *Starting Out in Rural Practice.* Department of Social and Administrative Medicine, University of North Carolina at Chapel Hill, 1980.
13. Eisenberg B, Cantwell J: Policies to influence the spatial distribution of physicians: A conceptual review of selected programs and empirical evidence. *Medical Care* 14:455–468, 1976.

14. Schwartz W, Newhouse J, Bennett B, et al: The changing geographic distribution of board-certified physicians. *New England Journal of Medicine* 303:1032–1037, 1980.

15. Geographic distribution of board-certified physicians, letter. *New England Journal of Medicine* 304:916–917, 1981.

16. Davis K, Marshall R: Primary health care services for medically underserved populations, in: *Papers on the National Health Guidelines: The Priorities of Section 1502.* USDHEW, Health Resources Administration, 1977.

17. Hassinger E, Hobbs D: The relation of community context to utilization of health services in a rural area. *Medical Care* 11:509–522, 1973.

18. Aday L, Andersen R, Fleming G: *Health Care in the U.S.—Equitable for Whom?* Beverly Hills, Calif, Sage Publications, 1980.

19. Kennedy V: Locational aspects of medical care-seeking in a rural population, with some implications for public policy research. *Journal of Health Politics, Policy and Law* 5:142–151, 1980.

20. Wright D: Recent rural health research. *Journal of Community Health* 1:60–72, 1976.

21. Kane R, Westover P: Rural health care research: Past accomplishments and future challenges. *Health Care Dimensions* 3:123–134, 1976.

22. Watkins J, Watkins D: Considerations in creating rural health care centers. *Journal of Family and Community Health* 2:85–94, 1979.

23. Rockoff M, Gorin L, Kleinman J: Positive programming—The use of data in planning for the rural health initiative. *Journal of Community Health* 4:204–216, 1979.

24. *Progress and Problems in Improving the Availability of Primary Care Providers in Underserved Areas.* U.S. General Accounting Office, 1978.

25. O'Leary J, Barton S: Health cooperatives in rural communities. *Bioscientific Communications* 3:218–230, 1977.

26. Sheps C, Bachar M: Rural areas and personal health services: Current strategies. *American Journal of Public Health* 71(suppl):71–82, 1981.

27. *Health Care Delivery in Rural Areas.* Chicago, American Medical Association, 1976.

28. Kane R, Warnick R, Proctor P, et al: Mail-Order medicine—An analysis of the Sears Roebuck Foundation's community medical assistance program. *Journal of the American Medical Association* 232:1023–1027, 1975.

29. Kane R: Problems in rural health care, in: *Health Services: The Local Perspective.* New York, Academy of Political Science, 1977.

30. Golladay F, Koch-Weser C: The new policies for rural health: Institu-

tional, social, and financial challenges to large-scale implementation. *Proceedings of the Royal Society of London Series B* 199:169–178, 1977.

31. Cowen D, Hochstrasser D, Fredericks C, Payne J: Problems in the development of a rural primary care center. *Journal of Community Health* 2:52–59, 1976.

32. Reilly B, Legge J, Reilly M: A rural health perspective: Principles for rural health policy. *Inquiry* 17:120–127, 1980.

33. Sorensen A, Parker R: Rural practices: Establishment by foreign medical graduates. *New York State Journal of Medicine* 54:1965–1966, 1978.

34. Rosenblatt R, Moscovice I: Establishing new rural family practices: Some lessons from a federal experience. *Journal of Family Practice* 7:755–763, 1978.

35. Appalachian Regional Commission Health Staff Presentation: Toward a rural health policy. Presented at American Public Health Association Annual Meeting, New York, October, 1977.

36. Onion D, Conant C, Dixon D, et al: Rural health care: A case study in Maine. *Medical Group Management*, 17–24, July 1980.

37. Wallack S, Kretz S: *Rural Medicine: Obstacles and Solutions for Self-Sufficiency.* Lexington, Mass, Lexington Books, 1981.

38. Madison D: Recruiting physicians for rural practice. *Health Services Reports* 88:758–762, 1973.

39. Kane R, Olsen D, Wright D, et al: Changes in utilization patterns in a national health service corps community. *Medical Care* 16:828–836, 1978.

40. Reynolds R, Banks S, Murphee A: *The Health of a Rural County.* Gainesville, University of Florida Press, 1976.

41. Geyman J (ed): Content of family practice—A statewide study in Virginia with its clinical, educational, and research implications. *Journal of Family Practice* 3:23–68, 1976.

42. Geyman J: Hospital practice of the family physician. *Journal of Family Practice* 8:911–912, 1979.

43. Slabaugh R, Ringiewicz M, Babineau R: The hospital work of a family practice group in a medium sized community in New England. *Journal of Family Practice* 11:287–297, 1980.

44. Nickerson R, Colton T, Peterson O, et al: Doctors who perform operations. *New England Journal of Medicine* 295:921–926, 1976.

45. Kane R, Olsen D, Newman J, et al: Giving and getting surgery in Utah: An urban-rural comparison. *Surgery* 83:373–381, 1978.

46. Reinhardt U: *Physician Productivity and the Demand for Health Manpower.* Cambridge, Mass, Ballinger, 1975.

47. Evashwick C: The role of group practice in the distribution of physicians in nonmetropolitan areas. *Medical Care* 14:808–823, 1976.

48. Scheffler, R: Productivity and economies of scale in medical practice,

in Rafferty J (ed): *Health Manpower and Productivity.* Lexington, Mass, Lexington Books, 1974.

49. Luft H: HMO performance: Current knowledge and questions for the 1980's. *The Group Health Journal,* 34–40, Winter 1980.

50. Somers A, Somers H: *Health and Health Care—Policies in Perspective.* Germantown, Aspen Systems Corp., Germantown, Maryland, 1977.

51. Held P, Reinhardt U (eds): *Analysis of Economic Performance in Medical Group Practices.* Final Report of Mathematica Policy Research for NCHSR Contract #HRA–106–74–0119, 1979.

52. Feldman R, Deitz D, Brooks E: The financial viability of rural primary health care centers. *American Journal of Public Health* 68:981–987, 1978.

53. Mechanic D, Greenleg J, Cleary P, et al: A model of rural health care: Consumer response among users of the Marshfield Clinic. *Medical Care* 18:597–608, 1980.

54. Konrad T, Johnson J, Madison D, Tilson H: Physician staff recruitment in large practice organizations—Part 1. *Medical Group Management* 23:12–20, 43, 1976.

55. Christianson J: Consumer preference for group practice medical services in rural areas. *Journal of Consumer Affairs* 14:418–433, 1980.

56. Cotterill P, Eisenberg B: Improving access to medical care in underserved areas: The role of group practice. *Inquiry* 16:141–153, 1979.

57. Glenn J, Hofmeister R: Will physicians rush out and get physician extenders. *Health Services Research* 11:69–74, 1976.

58. Wilson G: Productivity and the economics of primary care, in Noble J (ed): *Primary Care and the Practice of Medicine.* Boston, Little, Brown and Co., 1976.

59. Glenn J, Goldman J: Strategies for productivity with physician extenders. *Western Journal of Medicine* 124:249–257, 1976.

60. Record J, McCalley M, Schweitzer S, et al: New health professionals after a decade and a half: Delegation, productivity, and costs in primary care. *Journal of Health Politics, Policy and Law* 5:470–497, 1980.

61. Lawrence D: The impact of physician assistants and nurse practitioners on health care access, costs, and quality: A review of the literature. *Health and Medical Care Services Review* 1:1–12, 1978.

62. Kane R, Wilson W: The new health practitioners—The past as prologue. *Western Journal of Medicine* 127:254–261, 1977.

63. Cherkin D: Factors influencing the physician market for primary care new health practitioners. *Medical Care* 18:1097–1113, 1980.

64. Golladay F, et al: Policy planning for the mid-level health worker: Economic potentials and barriers to change. *Inquiry* 13:80–89, 1976.

65. Rosenblatt R, Moscovice I: The growth and evolution of rural primary care practice—The National Health Services Corps experience in the Northwest. *Medical Care* 16:819–827, 1978.

66. Moscovice I, Rosenblatt R: Rural health care delivery amidst federal retrenchment: Lessons from the Robert Wood Johnson Foundation's Rural Practice Project. *American Journal of Public Health*, forthcoming.

67. Call R, Howard M: Rural health—A three pronged approach. *Clinical Medicine* 83:9–13, 1976.

68. Block J: Hospital innovations in the community: Ambulatory care. *Bulletin of the New York Academy of Medicine* 55:104–111, 1979.

69. Gold M: Hospital based versus free-standing primary care costs. *Journal of Ambulatory Care Management* 2:1–20, 1979.

70. Saward E: The current role of the hospital in ambulatory care. *Bulletin of the New York Academy of Medicine* 55:112–118, 1979.

71. Madison D, Bernstein J: Special problems of primary care in rural areas, in: *Community Hospitals and the Challenge of Primary Care.* New York, Center for Community Health Systems, Columbia University, January 1975.

72. Shortell S, Dowling W, Urban N, et al: Hospital sponsored primary care: Organizational and financial issues. *Medical Group Management* 25:16,18,20–21,66, 1978.

73. Williams S, Wickizer T, Shortell S: Hospital-based ambulatory care—A national survey. Hospital and Health Services Administration. 26:66–80, 1981.

74. Green B: Rural health delivery systems of the 1980's. *Journal of Family and Community Health* 2:95–108, 1979.

75. Lewis C: Health maintenance organizations: Guarantors of access to medical care, in Lewis C, Fein R, Mechanic D: *A Right to Health.* New York, John Wiley and Sons, 1976.

76. Personal communication with HMO Office, USDHHS, 1981.

77. National Health Standards and Quality Information Clearinghouse: *Information Bulletin: Rural Health Care.* Baltimore, HCFA, 1980.

78. Hillis F, Miller W: Need, not numbers: The rural HMO. *New England Journal of Medicine* 291:580–581, 1974.

79. Nycz G, Wenzel F, Lohrenz F, et al: Composition of the subscribers in a rural prepaid group practice plan. *Public Health Reports* 91:504–507, 1976.

80. Averill B: Planning and developing an HMO in a semirural community, in *Management and Policy Issues in HMO Development.* Washington, DC, GHAA, 1979.

81. Federacion Rural de Salud de California—Advocate for the Health Care Needs of Rural Poor, mimeo, Fresno, 1978.

82. Newton A: Rural health care thrives under hospital's prepaid plan. *Hospitals* 51:45–48, 1977.

83. Lennie J: Economic viability of community operated prepaid health plan. *Health Care Management Review* 1:53–57, 1976.

84. Leitch C, Mitchell E: A state by state report: The legal accommodation of nurses practicing expanded roles. *Nurse Practitioner* 2:19–22, 1977.
85. Kissam P: Physician assistant and nurse practitioner laws for expanded medical delegation, in Bliss A, Cohen E (eds): *New Health Professionals.* Germantown, Aspen Systems Corp., Germantown, Maryland, 1977.
86. Bernstein J, Brooks E, De Friese G: Rural health services—Studies of workable models. Paper presented at American Public Health Association Annual Meeting, New York, October, 1977.
87. Schweitzer S, Record J: Third party payments for new health professionals: An alternative to federal reimbursement in outpatient care. *Public Health Reports* 92:518–526, 1977.
88. Moscovice I, Rosenblatt R: The viability of mid-level practitioners in isolated rural communities. *American Journal of Public Health* 69:503–505, 1979.
89. *New Health Professionals: Their Place in Primary Care.* Health Services Research Center, University of North Carolina. Chapel Hill, 1977.
90. Rosenblatt R, Huard B: The nurse practitioner as a physician substitute in a remote rural community: A case study. *Public Health Reports* 94:571–575, 1979.
91. LeRoy L, Lee P: *Deliberations and Compromise: The Health Professions Educational Assistance Act of 1976.* Cambridge, Mass, Ballinger, 1977.
92. Rosenblatt R, Moscovice I: The National Health Service Corps: Rapid growth and uncertain future. *Milbank Memorial Fund Quarterly* 58:282–309, 1980.
93. Sussman G, Steinfeldt L: Capacity building, linkages and rural health systems: The federal perspective. *Public Health Reports* 96:50–57, 1981.
94. Davis K, Gold M, Makuc D: Access to health care for the poor: Does the gap remain? *Annual Review of Public Health*, Palo Alto, Annual Reviews Inc., Volume 2, 1981, pp 159–183.
95. California Rural Health Federation: *A Band-Aid for Pancho.* Position Paper, Fresno, 1977.
96. Ahearn M: *Health Care in Rural America.* Agriculture Information Bulletin No. 428. US Department of Agriculture, 1979.
97. Roemer, M: *Rural Health Care.* St. Louis, C. V. Mosby Company, 1976.
98. Tilson H, Jellinek P: Primary health care and the local health department: The North Carolina experience. *American Journal of Public Health* 71(suppl):35–45, 1981.
99. Miller CA, Moos M, Kotch J, et al: Role of health departments in the delivery of ambulatory care. *American Journal of Public Health* 71(suppl):15–29, 1981.

CHAPTER 5

Rural Emergency Medical Care

Emergency! The sudden onset of a life-threatening condition, either through injury or acute illness, is at the same time commonplace and profoundly unsettling. Societies have special rules for the response to emergencies; laws are passed that recognize the protected status of the layman or professional who goes to the aid of the acutely injured or disabled person. Awards are given for unusual heroism in responding to someone in need of emergency attention. Institutions like the Red Cross orient themselves around their ability to offer help to communities struck by emergencies.

Rural communities are particularly susceptible to the effects of emergencies. As discussed in Chapter 3, some rural professions carry with them a much higher incidence of accidental injury. These include logging, farming, and fruit picking. Injuries account for a significant proportion of all rural health care visits—over 17 percent of all visits were for trauma in one study.[1] The scattered nature of rural settlement can transform a routine accident into a potential tragedy. The injured worker may not be discovered soon, and when the worker is discovered, help may be remote. Even when assistance is called, the emergency resources may be meager and the trip to definitive care long.

For these reasons, emergency medical services are of particular interest to rural communities. In many cases, the intense desire of a rural community for local medical professionals stems from its desire for adequate emergency care. In fact, rural dwellers may use local providers only in emergencies and not use them when obtaining routine or scheduled medical care. However, as we will explore in this chapter, an adequate emergency care system must be built on the foundation of an efficient and ongoing conventional medical care system. As in the field of rural health care in general, each service must be integrated with every other service in order to maintain the financial integrity and technical proficiency of the system.

In the development of a rural health care system, the emergency service component should receive priority. Although we have demonstrated the disruptive societal effect on a community of not having primary medical services readily available, these are usually not life-threatening deficiencies. In most American communities, the major consequences of unavailable ambulatory services are wasted time and money due to the necessity to travel to remote communities for routine medical care. This of course has a deleterious effect on the community itself, raises the cost of medical care by introducing the burden of travel, and, probably, yields a lower quality of medical care simply because the cultural and spatial distance between provider and client is greater. It is in the emergency situation that the consequence is immediate and critical. Although truly life-threatening emergencies are not everyday events, they are not rare. Automobile and occupational accidents are a predictable part of life, and in specific instances, the speed and proficiency of the medical response have a direct impact on life or death, recovery, or disability.

Rural residents are susceptible to the failure of the system to respond to emergency situations. As Waller points out, "for most types of injury resulting in death, those injured in rural areas (as compared to urban areas) more frequently die in the first hour."[2] This increased death rate is due not to the increased severity of injury in rural areas, but because of the generally delayed response to that emergency by the health care system. "Rural residents themselves have emergencies that, potentially or actually, are more serious than those of urban residents. . . . Residents of individual rural counties are in some cases more than ten times as likely to die of their injury as their urban counterparts."[2] The increased rate of injuries in rural areas and the higher likelihood of death as an outcome is also echoed by Kane and his co-writers in their review of rural health research.[3]

Organized systems of emergency care are relatively recent developments in American health care. Only over the last 20 years has there been the realization that effective prehospital care of emergency victims should be systematically handled by trained personnel. The military experiences of the Korean and Viet Nam Wars illustrated the dramatic decrease in mortality that could be achieved by rapid response of skilled personnel with appropriate equipment, even under adverse battlefield conditions. The medical technology developed during these conflicts was immediately transferred to the civilian sector. Injuries and deaths generated by the proliferation of automobiles offered many situations in which these new skills could be utilized. Substantial private and government investment has been funneled into emergency health care, particularly in the last 10 years. This has transformed totally both the concept and the practice of emergency medical care.

The disparity between urban and rural standards of health care is particularly apparent in emergency medical services (EMS). Because emergencies are unpredictable, emergency health care systems are by definition underused. In the densely populated urban area, the volume of demand is adequate to support a full-time professional emergency care apparatus, bridging the spectrum from emergency dispatch systems to emergency medical technicians, paramedics, emergency-room physicians, and all the commensurate technology. In rural areas, it is economically impossible to support the ponderous weight of a full-time professional EMS system. It is no accident that the majority of ambulance systems in rural areas were run until relatively recently by funeral parlors. The rationale behind using funeral homes and their personnel for emergency medical services was that funeral services, just like emergency medical services, were relatively infrequently needed in rural areas. The rationale remains intact today. The rural emergency medical care system cannot afford to stand apart as a paid, single-purpose professional entity. Rural emergency care functions must be built upon existing medical institutions and personnel, as well as volunteers. It is a dismal reflection on the relative ineffectiveness of the old emergency medical care response capability that the undertaker inherited the socially anointed role of picking up the dead and injured.

In this chapter, we will review the recent explosive developments in the field of emergency health care in the country at large and the impact of these changes in rural America. We will then discuss the elements of emergency medical care in an attempt to identify those aspects in which improvements have a demonstrable effect on the health and well being of the population. Next, we will discuss the various elements of the system that must be developed, review some of the recent efforts in rural communities to meet the very real barriers to establishing effective rural emergency medical care systems, and recommend a plausible approach towards the development of such a system that is professionally and financially justified.

HISTORICAL DEVELOPMENT OF EMERGENCY MEDICAL CARE SYSTEMS

The current configuration of emergency medical services systems (EMS) is the product of an intense set of public and private activities over a very short period of time. EMS activities before 1960 were almost entirely ad hoc local responses of limited utility. If the core function of an EMS system is to avert death and disability by the quick and effective treatment of the injured and ill, then EMS was, until recently, a failure. The major function of the ambulance services—the symbolic core of those EMS systems that existed—was patient transport. Patients with life-threatening disease or injury whose lives could have been salvaged died of benign neglect, usually while being transported from the scene of an accident to the nearest hospital.

The rapid growth of the EMS system is a rather unusual example of technological advance and political innovation acting in tandem. As mentioned before, military experience generated a rapid advance in the capacity of the medical care system to care for the critically injured. In the mid-1960s, it became widely recognized and publicized that there was a large gap between what was being done and what was possible in the field of EMS. The first major government intervention occurred in 1966 when the National Highway Safety Act established an EMS branch and allotted funds to plan and implement some experimental EMS systems around the country.[4]

The establishment of a limited number of integrated EMS

systems—systems including central dispatch, radio communications, treatment protocols, hospital categorization, standing orders, and coordination of providers—made the disparity between what was achievable and what was being done increasingly obvious. In the 1970s, a number of foundations made major commitments to EMS development, and in 1973 the intense ferment around EMS culminated in the Emergency Medical Systems Act of 1973 (PL 93–154), a remarkably comprehensive body of legislation that established uniform criteria for an adequate EMS system and made available funds for local, regional, and state governments to build both basic and advanced EMS systems.

The rapid infusion of money into a fairly undeveloped area created a certain degree of confusion. As Andrews points out, "The availability of funds for upgrading EMS from various levels of government and private foundations has far exceeded the capacity to use such funds effectively."[5] Communities realized that EMS was a high priority and became aware that funds were available to purchase much of the glamorous and expensive equipment—ambulances, communications equipment, defribrillators—that were the status symbols of this new game. However, there often was little basic understanding of which elements of the system were really necessary to avert death and what were the fiscal and organizational consequences of building elaborate EMS systems in areas that might not be able to maintain them.

The 1973 EMS act was in itself a very useful educational vehicle for those communities who applied for funds under its provisions. The law defined an acceptable EMS system on the basis of 15 interlocking components that ranged from facilities and mutual aid agreements, to the selection and training of paramedical personnel, to policies that insured consumer participation and adequate regional governance. In order to receive funds under the act, applicants had to demonstrate that they had considered each of the system's elements. Although in reality many of the EMS grants were focused on purchasing expensive hardware rather than on attaining some standard of acceptable function, communities were at least forced to consider the fact that a successful EMS system depended on attention to a wide spectrum of interlocking elements.

In its simplest form, the EMS act and its subsequent extensions and amendments have established two basic levels of emergency medical care capability. The first level, Basic Life Support (BLS), is built essentially on three major elements: personnel, emergency transport, and life-support equipment. The personnel that are the core of the system are designated as Emergency Medical Technicians at the starting, or "A" level (EMT-A's) individuals who have successfully completed an 81-hour-long training course originally developed by Dunlop Associates for the Department of Transportation (DOT). This 81-hour course presents the rudimentary theoretical base of emergency medical care and gives the EMT basic skills in the recognition, stabilization, and transport of critically ill or injured people. EMT-A's can be professional ambulance attendants, policemen, firemen, community volunteers, or other individuals, and this level of training is designed to be a base upon which additional knowledge and skills can be added.

In the Basic Life Support system, the EMTs use an ambulance meeting quite rigorous DOT standards and equipped according to guidelines set down by the American College of Surgeons. These EMTs, with their equipment, have the theoretical capacity to respond appropriately to the bulk of emergency situations that arise. The effectiveness of their response will depend to a large degree on the quality of the system, the location of the ambulances, the frequency of continuing education and review, the enthusiasm of the public sponsoring body, and the economic solvency of the entire system. These elements will be discussed in more detail later.

The second level is the Advanced Life Support (ALS) system. The core characteristic of the BLS system is rapid transport of the injured person to a location where definitive therapy can be given. It is essentially a passive system with regard to the disease process afflicting the patient. ALS is designed to make available to the victim personnel who can actively intervene to maintain life or prevent life-threatening sequelae of the initial process. In ALS, the EMT is replaced by the paramedic, whose training typically involves from 500 to 2,000 hours of classroom and supervised clinical training. These individuals are capable of initiating intravenous therapy, giving drugs—usually while consulting with physicians by radio—establishing an airway, and using defibrillators after obtaining and assessing electrocardiograms. The transport vehicles resemble mobile intensive care units, and the amount of equipment parallels that of many an emergency room. These sophisticated and expensive systems exist in a number of urban areas throughout the country and have diffused into a few rural areas as well.

These two levels provide benchmarks against which we can assess the adequacy of rural EMS systems. Paradoxically, it is in rural areas—with long transport times, and, often, marginally staffed hospitals—where advanced life support is most needed and least available. As Boyd has commented, "While most of the activity in the ALS system is currently in metropolitan areas, an appreciation of the need for ALS and critical care services for the rural and outlying areas is now developing. A national goal will be to realize these essential emergencies and critical care services of the rural emergency patient at the scene and during the long transportation periods to distant appropriate treatment facilities."[6]

Through the more than 300 regional EMS districts established under the federal Emergency Medical Systems Act, there has been a total transformation of emergency medical care in the country, in both rural and urban areas. However, rural emergency care is still in a period of rapid evolution, and we are in an excellent position to learn and generalize from the many demonstrations and experiments that have occurred in the last five years. The rest of this chapter will deal specifically with the conceptual framework within whch planning for emergency care must proceed and apply this specifically to the rural situation.

EMERGENCY MEDICAL CARE— A CONCEPTUAL FRAMEWORK

The term *emergency* has two major connotations. First, any given emergency is unpredictable. Second, an emergency demands prompt intervention. A medical emergency usually occurs suddenly and unexpectedly and is of such severity that an immediate response is necessary.

True medical emergencies are uncommon events in the life of an individual. Most illness proclaims itself slowly, allowing the patient sufficient time to seek medical care through routine channels. Most cases that find their way to emergency rooms or are handled by emergency medical systems are also not truly urgent. Although there is considerable variation in the reported figures, observers estimate that only five percent of those entering into the EMS system are critical,[6] and only 1.5 percent of those cared for in emergency rooms are in a critical condition. Yet it is this tip of the iceberg, this five percent, for whom the emergency care system ostensibly exists.

The quintessential example of an emergency is a major injury. Mechanisms to deal with injury, whether generated by natural disaster, military misadventure, or occupational mishap, have been a part of our cultural expectations for generations. However, an epidemiological theory that explains the occurrence of injury in a cohesive way is a fairly recent development. Haddon and others, working over the last 40 years, have explored the notion that injuries are best understood in a manner analogous to our comprehension of infectious disease. Injuries are the results of destructive energies applied to a susceptible host. The energy may be mechanical, thermal, chemical, radiologic, or the like; the host's susceptibility is a product of genetics, physiological status, location, inherent and acquired resistance, and other factors. Using this metaphor, it is possible logically to catalogue and approach different types of injuries and begin to analyze why they occur and how they can be prevented.[7]

The concept of an emergency due to physical illness can also be understood in this fashion. Infectious, mechanical, chemical, and electrical malfunctions within the individual lead to sudden and catastrophic disruption in normal physiological function. Injuries and illness differ mostly in the time scale involved. Injuries tend to cause their destructive effects within very brief amounts of time—typically less than a second—while emergent disease is usually the product of a chronic although often subclinical process. In both cases, prevention must be a major focus, although the mechanisms of prevention are much more concrete in the case of physical injury.[8]

The basic rationale for an emergency medical care system is that rapid intervention can ameliorate or prevent disease or disability. It is important to examine this assumption critically before beginning to design any EMS system. Injuries and diseases in which time is not a factor, as well as injuries or diseases not amenable to useful intervention, require a different type of response than those for which every moment counts. We must identify those conditions where timely intervention makes a difference and design the system around those interventions.

It is useful to examine the pathophysiological consequences of disease or injuries that consign them to the class of emergencies. For example, airway obstruction is an emergency because the lack of oxygen leads to rapid brain death, and prompt intervention can prevent this outcome. Airway obstruction can occur as the result of trauma—for instance, a fracture of the jaw—or as the result of a disease process, such as swelling of the airway secondary to a bacterial infection. Both are emergencies requiring rapid and sophisticated intervention to prevent death or irreversible physiologic damage.

By identifying the final common physiological pathways for the majority of emergent conditions, we can begin to determine what the characteristics must be of an effective emergency medical system. In order to perform this analysis, it is useful to look at the time course of different elements of the emergency. First, we must determine the amount of time that elapses from the onset of symptoms to that point at which the patient's condition becomes critical, the symptom-to-criticality interval. This measures the rate of change of the severity of the condition and is largely determined by the biological nature of the emergency. The second measure is the time from the onset of symptoms until the first contact with the medical care system, the symptom-to-contact interval. This reflects the appraisal of the patient or those around the patient of the urgency of the condition, as well as access to some way of calling for help. The third measure is the time elapsing from time of notification to the moment when the first restorative intervention begins, the contact-to-intervention interval. This is a direct measure of both the efficiency and the capability of the EMS system, in terms of the speed at which an individual with the appropriate skills arrives at the patient's side and institutes treatment.

Figure 5.1 illustrates the fact that patients with critical illnesses who use the emergency medical care system can be divided into two distinct subpopulations. The first subpopulation consists of those whose disease or injury is not time sensitive and whose ultimate survival is not materially affected by the briskness of the emergency response. This group has two subpopulations, a smaller group in whom death is inevitable because of the massive nature of the insult to their physiological integrity, and a second group whose disorder, although critical, has a relatively leisurely time course. These latter patients can benefit from the transport and stabilization function of

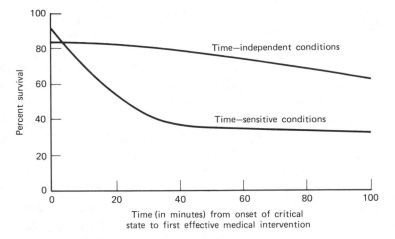

Figure 5.1. The effect of the rapidity of treatment on survival rate in two subpopulations. (Adapted from Figure 2 in Andrews, RB: Viewing EMS as a system. In: Emergency Medical Services Systems as a Health Services Research Setting. USDHEW, DHEW Pub. No. (PHS) 79–3233, 1978)

the EMS system, but rapid and heroic intervention is not required to save lives.

The second curve represents those patients whose conditions are time sensitive. Patient survival depends on the speed with which appropriate medical intervention is initiated. It is this group around which the emergency medical care system must be built and against which its effectiveness is measured.

Despite the rather obvious natures of these two subpopulations, we still have relatively little information about the relative size of these two patient subgroups, nor do we know as much as we would like about the effectiveness of the EMS system in making a difference in life-threatening disease. In one study, it was found that a very small proportion—as low as one in a thousand of all emergency patients—fall into the group whose "survival is highly dependent on the rapidity with which they receive restorative treatments."[5] Moreover, this group had certain other uniform characteristics: They contacted the EMS system within 15 minutes of the onset of symptoms, and they were largely savable if assistance reached them promptly. The major diagnoses in this group included disorders of cardiac rhythm and drownings, but not many trauma patients.

These data are somewhat startling in the small proportion of all patients whose conditions were time sensitive. In most cases handled by the emergency medical care system, the outcome is relatively independent of the time that elapses from the onset of symptoms to the point at which intervention begins. A small subset of individuals with specific disorders, such as a cardiac arrhythmia, do benefit from rapid treatment. A study of the very sophisticated Medic One system in Seattle appears to support this perception. In this study, the response time of the paramedic teams was not a factor in determining ultimate survival when all diagnoses were examined together.[9] However, when just those patients with cardiac arrest are considered separately, patient survival is enhanced by rapid paramedic response.[10] In any case, compared with the overwhelming importance of the baseline physiological state of the individual and the nature of the illness or injury, time becomes a relatively less important ingredient in survival.

As Figure 5.1 illustrates, however, there is definitely one segment of the population in which the survival rate can be doubled by rapid emergency response. It is also possible that as we improve the capability of emergency medical technicians to intervene in selected conditions, additional patients will fall into the time-sensitive subpopulation. Moreover, Figure 5.1 deals only with mortality rates. It is likely that an additional segment of the population has lower morbidity rates, fewer sequelae, and shorter hospital courses as the result of effective early emergency intervention.

Although the data are scanty, examining the actual physiological dimensions of the patient in need of emergency care allows us to begin to structure an EMS system. First, the system must be able to deal with a wide spectrum of patients who will enter it. Some of them will be massively, irrevocably injured, although it is often impossible to make that assessment when the patient is first encountered. A second rather small group will have conditions in which immediate intervention will save lives. The EMTs and paramedics who staff the EMS system must be trained to recognize these entities and initiate treatment. Since there is a definable group—albeit small—in which survival decreases rapidly with the time that elapses before help arises, it becomes particularly important that in rural areas those arriving first at the scene be capable of initiating appropriate treatment. It is ironic that the urban

paramedics are most likely to have the broad repertoire of emergency skills, whereas the rural EMT may have only rudimentary
training. It is in the rural area—not in the urban area, where most
victims are only minutes from a hospital—where a trained
emergency responder is likely to be able to save lives.

There is another important and problematic aspect of emergency care systems—the maintenance of adequate skills among
the EMS personnel. The reality is that the vast majority of emergency cases seen in the rural and urban areas do not require sophisticated emergency skills on the part of the emergency responder.
A basic problem of providing adequate emergency care in the
rural area is that even the well-trained responder will rarely encounter a situation that will utilize his hard-earned skills. Therefore,
any rural emergency medical care system will require highly motivated individuals willing to devote considerable energy to acquiring
and maintaining skills in order to assure that the system will be
competent to deal with frequent but critical events.

THE MAJOR COMPONENTS OF A RURAL MEDICAL SYSTEM

There are five components of a rural emergency medical care
system that warrant in-depth discussion. They are personnel, transportation, communication, the role of the hospital, and the administrative framework. Although there are numerous ways to categorize
the elements of an emergency medical services system, these five
heterogeneous categories capture the essence of the system. If a
given EMS region has considered and solved the problems of assuring adequate preparation in each of these areas, the resulting EMS
response should be functional.

PERSONNEL

The purpose of the EMS system is to bring patients into contact
with trained emergency providers in a setting where the providers
can use their skills. Until very recently, this involved transporting

patients by ambulance or other conveyance to a hospital where therapy was initiated. In the hospital, physicians and nurses would begin the process of intervening into the basic pathophysiological process that initiated the emergency.

The single most important innovation of the EMS system has been to bring some of the skills of the physician and the nurse—and some of the equipment of the hospital—to the stricken patient. The rationale behind this transformation from a passive to an active system of outreach has been that earlier effective intervention improves outcome. This is clear in at least certain types of disease processes, and it is this observation that has provided the impetus for the transformation of the way emergency medical care is rendered in the United States.

This new system has created a new type of health provider, the emergency medical technician. To a large extent, the efficacy of the entire system depends upon the capability of this individual to meet the rather far-reaching expectations that fall upon him or her. We have discussed the two levels of training for EMTs, and thousands of rural Americans have become EMT-A's by successfully completing the standard 81-hour training program. To what extent does this adequately prepare them for the challenges of the job?

A study of 4,555 patients cared for by EMT-A's in Connecticut gives an informative but not entirely reassuring answer to that question.[11] The diagnostic accuracy of the EMTs—their ability to correctly assess and name the patient's problem—was mediocre; they frequently were unable to determine the true nature of the problem. Treatment appropriateness was more variable; they were much more adept at appropriately treating life-threatening or serious illness than nonserious conditions.

The implications of this study are that we should be cautious in our expectations of the EMS system. It is comforting to realize that the EMT-A's are best at doing that which is most critical—intervening in serious and life-threatening illness. Although their diagnostic abilities are poor, a diagnosis is not always required before initiating treatment. Since the response to many life-threatening illnesses is quite similar—establish an airway, restore circulation, stop blood loss, and replace blood volume—accurate diagnosis is often unnecessary.

By the same token, it is important that EMT-A's refrain from intervening in cases where immediate treatment is not needed. There is a very real tendency for EMTs to practice meddlesome emergency care, attempting to treat conditions that are better left to more definitive diagnostic and therapeutic maneuvers in a hospital emergency room. There are a number of conditions, such as head injury or pneumothorax, for which the wrong diagnosis and the wrong treatment can harm or kill the patient. There is definitely a place for continuing education for EMTs in an effort to improve their sophistication and comfort with a range of presenting emergency conditions.

There are very few advanced life-support systems operational in rural areas and only a handful of emergency responders trained to the stringent standards required of the EMTs that staff these systems. In some rural areas, nurse practitioners, physician's assistants, and physicians may themselves respond to certain kinds of emergencies, although it is usually impractical for them to go along on every ambulance call. A number of observers have emphasized the importance of a higher level of training for rural EMTs than that provided in the basic 81-hour course. As noted in the previous section, it is in areas where response times are long that it is most important that the person arriving in the ambulance be capable of instituting therapy. Yet, it is impractical to attempt to have significant numbers of rural EMTs—for the most part volunteers—attain the higher levels of training.

Spoor describes a program in rural New York state that directly addresses the problem of advanced training. Instead of attempting to give the entire paramedic training sequence to their EMTs, they broke the course up into smaller modules and presented them sequentially. They began with the intravenous (IV) therapy module, using specially designed anatomical simulations as training devices, and were able to attain a satisfactory success rate when the EMTs were called upon to start IVs under field conditions. They felt that it was more practical to teach the skills in a discontinuous fashion and not overwhelm their volunteer crews. They do comment however, "Unfortunately, most federal and state agencies still require that the training for rural ambulance services be modeled on that given in urban areas."[12] Since funding and reimbursement may be tied to certain levels of certification, this inflexibility may inhibit the natural evolution of emergency skills in rural EMS systems.

Waller also discusses in detail the essential importance of continued education in the maintenance of the skills of EMTs.[13] EMTs must retain their skills in a set number of conditions, whether or not they have an opportunity to use all of those skills in real-life field situations. Since emergencies are sporadic affairs, no given EMT will have an adequate field exposure to all requisite skills during any given period of time. Therefore, one component of the EMS system must be a well-integrated program of continuing education that includes periodic critiques of actual performance and simulation and practice sessions which refresh the basic emergency skills. One attractive suggestion that Waller makes is that urban centers with busy emergency departments accept rural EMTs for short, intense, periodic refreshers. This would be an excellent and invigorating way to immerse the rural EMT in a broad spectrum of emergency activities.

TRANSPORTATION

Transportation serves two functions in today's EMS system. First, it brings the emergency medical technician to the scene of the accident or illness, and second, transportation brings the victim to a hospital where definitive therapy can be administered. The same vehicle need not necessarily be used for both purposes, and some of the most innovative EMS systems in both rural and urban units separate the two functions. For example, in the Medic One system in Seattle discussed earlier, regular fire trucks are used to bring firemen to the injured person in life-threatening emergencies; since fire stations are uniformly dispersed around the urban area, the response time is extremely short, often less than five minutes from the time of the initial call to the time that therapy begins. Fifty percent of the firemen are trained as EMTs and can initiate emergency medical procedures; all are trained in advanced first aid.

A similar rural model has been established in Marquette County, Wisconsin. The county was able to purchase two emergency vans, and these were placed at appropriate locations within the rural county. EMTs, however, were selected based upon their dispersion throughout the county such that the EMTs were able to arrive at the scene of the accident or illness much more quickly than the vans. Each of the EMTs was supplied with a *jump kit*—a set of the basic devices to allow the initiation of therapy—and the EMTs and the vans were dispatched simultaneously by the sheriff's office. [14]

This dual response system is conceptually identical to the urban Medic One system. It has the advantage of insuring rapid response without excessive investment in relatively infrequently used ambulances. It has the disadvantage of being more administratively complex. However, the logic of the approach is compelling if it can be supported and maintained. There are obviously many potential variations on the theme, but the main point of the concept is to increase the speed of the response by getting the first responder to the scene without making him or her dependent on an ambulance for transportation.

Ambulance location also has a major impact on the average response time within the geographic area served by the ambulance. The real difficulty comes in trying to decide what capabilities the system should have. Because of the sparsely populated nature of rural areas, there is an inherent inefficiency in any ambulance service, since the ambulance will not be used the majority of the time. Therefore, it is important not to invest more money than necessary in buying and maintaining these expensive vehicles. However, if the area covered is relatively large, one vehicle may be quite distant from some of the points of the service area, resulting in slow response times.

To determine optimal location, one must decide on some response standard; for example, the system should be able to respond to 95 percent of the calls within 30 minutes. Using this standard, it is then possible to decide how many ambulances are needed for the service area and where they should be placed. At the same time, one must determine the projected demand for ambulance services and determine what the probability is of receiving a call for assistance while the ambulance is already being used. In rural areas, demand overlap is relatively unlikely to occur, but expectations in this regard need to be explicit parts of the model.

A number of investigators have used this sort of static location model to plan ambulance services. [15-17] The demand for ambulance services is lower in rural areas, and this yields a relatively high cost for each ambulance run. As Daberkow points out, "It is obviously unrealistic to plan EMS systems around predetermined goals or standards without detailed considerations of the costs of

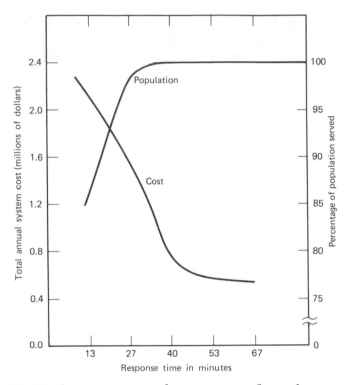

Figure 5.2. EMS system cost and percentage of population served as functions of ambulance response time. (Figure 2, Daberkow SG: Location and cost of ambulances serving a rural area. *Health Services Research*, Fall 1977.)

meeting them."[17] It is all very well to fashion a pristine mathematical model for rural ambulance services, but if the investment draws off resources that are needed for other parts of the health care system, the total effect may be negative. Figure 5.2 shows the relationship between total system cost and the response time standard; the more rapid the desired response, the more expensive the system.

    One important result of the analysis of the economic characteristics of rural ambulance systems is that they are relatively expensive and unlikely to be able to become self-supporting on the basis of fees generated from patients. A number of studies have been done on typical rural ambulance systems, and all indicate that they require substantial external subsidy. One major conclusion is that rural ambulance systems must be manned by volunteers or by policemen or others whose basic salary comes from another source. It is economically unfeasible to expect to be able to support a professional ambulance corps. Even in urban areas, these systems require substantial public subsidy; in rural areas, even with volunteer attendants, operational costs far exceed service-generated revenues. Doeksen et al. in a discussion of the expected costs under four different alternative ambulance systems, calculate that even with the least expensive system, an 80 percent subsidy—amounting to $50,000 per ambulance annually—is required.[18]

Ambulances are not the only vehicles used to transport the ill and the injured. Helicopters and fixed-wing aircraft are used widely in different parts of the country for emergency transport. They tend to be used in areas such as Alaska, where distances are enormous and highways are either rudimentary or nonexistent. They also have found a use as secondary transport vehicles where severely injured but relatively stable individuals are transported long distances for definitive care at specialized centers. Burn therapy is an example: injured soldiers are frequently flown from Europe to the United States for their medical care. Neonatal transport to neonatal intensive care units in special transport isolettes also occurs in multiple regionalized systems throughout the country.

Although a number of studies have shown the medical feasibility of using air transportation in emergency medical services,[19-21] the extremely high cost of this mode of transport makes it generally impractical to plan entire EMS systems around aircraft. The solutions that seem to work best are those in which helicopters and other aircraft are operated by government units for other primary functions but can be called upon in special situations to serve an EMS purpose. Excellent examples are the MAST system of the armed services and a variety of agreements calling upon the helicopter capability of the state patrol.[22] In these systems, the helicopters are used primarily for military or police duties but can be called upon by civilians for use in emergency transport. The cost is borne by the unit owning and operating the helicopters, and the marginal cost of using the aircraft for emergency transport is relatively modest.

Even in these situations, use of aircraft is not entirely without problems. Frequently, armed services units may be operated by reserve personnel, and they may be relatively inexperienced in emergency transport. In addition, given the various administrative units involved, it sometimes can require remarkably long periods of time to deploy aircraft such that the actual flight time becomes a fraction of the response time. In addition, not all aircraft are equipped for medical transport; many are cramped, noisy, and occasionally unstable, making it difficult to adequately monitor the patient's condition in flight.

In general, ambulance service will be the backbone of the rural emergency medical care system. Aircraft backup should be used if available, but those cases in which it will be used should be defined and organized in advance. In addition, those responsible for operating the system should not be dazzled by the technology and allure of the more expensive but less reliable systems. Given the inherent economic deficit built into EMS services, attention should be paid to creating the simplest, most foolproof system available.

COMMUNICATIONS

Communication devices are used during four different stages in the response of the emergency medical system. First, the communications component must enable any potential user to contact quickly a designated individual who can mobilize the emergency response. Second, the dispatch coordinator needs to be able to communicate with the personnel who will actually travel to the person in need. Third, the ambulance crew must be able to contact the hospital to which the patient will be taken, the backup physician, and other ambulances and hospitals during the period of patient transport. Fourth, the hospitals within the system must have a simple way of contacting other hospitals and ambulances within the system.

This is a complex part of the system, made more complex because it requires the successful integrating of different types of communications technology and the cooperation of a variety of people. Four ingredients are necessary for the communications system to successfully perform its mission: standardization of technology, centralization, coordination between regions, and ingenuity, with ingenuity being perhaps the most important component in small rural areas.

The communications system begins when someone sees an emergency situation and summons aid. In most cases, this is by telephone, and the 911 telephone systems of urban areas have greatly improved both the rapidity and appropriateness of the response. Thus, the first element of the communication system is having someone to call who can initiate an effective response.

In rural areas, 911 systems are technically and economically impracticable. In one small town, a substitute 911 system was designed in which one emergency number rang simultaneously in five locations: the local medical clinic, the physician's house, the nurse's house, and at the homes of two volunteers.[23] Each of these individuals was able to dispatch the volunteer EMTs and thus represented the rural equivalent of a 911 operator. Such a system, ingenious in its design and simplicity, depends on the dedication of those people manning the phone and is not entirely foolproof. However, it does illustrate what can be done by a volunteer system.

The problem is frequently complicated in rural areas by antiquated phone systems or a patchwork of disparate phone companies serving the same geographic areas. It is still not uncommon for rural areas to have multiparty lines, and neighbors must develop conventions that allow them to intrude into normal telephone calls for emergency reasons. More troublesome is the situation in which adjoining rural towns may be separated by a long-distance telephone charge. Although this will not inhibit use of the system in the true emergency, it can cause hesitation in the uncertain case. Only through continued improvement of rural phone systems will these barriers be removed.

The second link in the chain of communications is the response to the call, usually by dispatch of an ambulance or a volunteer EMT to the source of the call. A successful dispatch coordinator must have some rudimentary ability to triage calls, to differentiate between the totally frivolous and the truly urgent request. In addition, the dispatcher must be tied into the response system. He must know who is available to respond to calls, where they are currently located, and be able to get in touch with them. Increasingly, this last step is handled through some sort of paging system in which the volunteer aides carry portable voice pagers that can be signaled by the dispatcher.

The dispatch function requires that someone be constantly available at a central phone number; in most rural communities, the local sheriff or police station and the hospital are the two existing agencies with a 24-hour-a-day capacity to respond. The local law enforcement agency in general maintains an ongoing dispatch function and has the communications equipment needed to contact ambulances and their crews, as well as to link up with other communication systems outside their jurisdiction. The hospital is more likely to have personnel who are knowledgeable about the medical content of the emergency and to alert the ambulance crew to the type of situation they will be confronting. Small rural hospitals are often sparsely staffed during night shifts and thus may be overloaded by having to assume a major dispatch function. However, both solutions are widely used, and the system actually chosen will depend on the particular local circumstances that prevail.

Other ingenious solutions to this problem exist. The volunteer 911 system described above is one example. In some communities, other commercial paging systems set up by industries or businesses in the areas may be able to handle medical dispatch for low additional marginal costs. In one town in the state of Washington, a man crippled by a double amputation was established as a central dispatcher for the county by some of the local physicians. Starting with a system that was oriented to the needs of the local doctors who were sharing night calls, his service has now expanded to include a large commercial radio paging operation. Whichever system is devised, it must be continuous and reliable, and the quality is dependent on the common sense of the dispatcher at the end of the telephone.

The third step is a mobile radio system whereby the ambulance crew can communicate with the hospital and the physicians. This requires two-way radios with frequencies reserved for emergency communications. The importance of this particular link in the communication chain has increased with the upgrading of the skills of the ambulance attendants. EMTs with some advanced life-support skills intervene actively in a number of situations; they often need to consult immediately with a physician or nurse at the hospital who is familiar with the selection and dosages of drugs, such as in situations requiring administration of agents that stabilize cardiac rhythm. In rural areas, particularly in those with mountainous topography, the technology needed to connect remote parts of the county can be solved by the establishment of carefully placed repeaters on strategic hills. It is in this area that the FCC regulations that stipulate types of equipment and specific radio frequencies have brought some hope of uniformity in a chaotic field.[4]

The fourth function that the communications system should be capable of carrying out is contacting and exchanging information with resources outside of the immediate EMS area. In more densely settled areas, ambulances frequently will bypass certain hospitals in favor of hospitals with greater capacity to handle the particular problem. Although such hospital triage is ill advised in rural hospitals—as we will discuss below—at times ambulances will not carry patients to the usual home-base hospital. Instances also arise when additional vehicles are involved in a particular case, such as a transfer from an ambulance to an aircraft, then back to ambulance, and finally to a hospital—a not infrequent occurrence with severe injuries in remote areas. In these cases, communication devices must be compatible, or else there must be a central coordinating unit with the capacity to receive and broadcast on a variety of wavelengths.

This necessity for regional EMS systems to be able to communicate with each other mandates carefully planned and mutually agreed upon communications covenants at the state or multistate level. Spurred on by the EMS legislation and the bewildering array of mismatched communications systems that had evolved, many states have begun the painful, expensive process of imposing logic in communications. Nebraska, for example, went through a 10-year process of evaluating its telecommunication needs, establishing a coordinating agency at the state level to implement the recommendations, and enacting the legislation needed to force the process to happen. The resulting system has very sophisticated capabilities that build upon but also go beyond the needs of an EMS system and virtually tie the entire state together in a medical telecommunications network.[24] The process of accomplishing such radical change is protracted, painful, and expensive, but going through it helps introduce rationality and interchange throughout the entire system.

THE RURAL HOSPITAL AND EMERGENCY MEDICAL SERVICES

The hospital is the focal point and the anchor of the emergency medical system. The hospital is the distillation of the community's formal, ongoing commitment to medical care; it is the one institution in the rural community with the organizational and professional capability to plan, organize, and deliver a wide variety of health services. In certain select instances, a doctor's office or medical clinic takes on some of the broader functions usually assumed by hospitals. But in the general case, only the hospital has the administrative breadth and stability upon which a system can be built.

The rapid improvement in the prehospital phase of emergency medical care has underlined both the crucial importance and frequent inadequacy of the rural hospital emergency room. In the days before EMTs riding in well equipped ambulances became the established standard of care, most seriously impaired victims did not survive the trip to the emergency room. Now that the EMTs are maintaining life in this class of patients, it has become clear that inadequate or inappropriate response in the emergency room results in unnecessary death. In a Vermont study cited by Waller, approximately 23 percent of 162 persons injured died of injuries that were probably survivable using the resources already available in the rural setting. Half of the unnecessary deaths were attributed to the hospital phase of care, both in the emergency room and in later phases of care.[25]

We must therefore insure that the rural emergency room is capable of expeditiously and expertly handling those emergency cases that arrive on its doorstep, night or day. The key to developing this capability is well-trained personnel. In most rural emergency rooms, doctors are rarely available on the hospital premises. Initial stabilization and resuscitation are the responsibility of regular hospital staff, who must hold the fort until the physician arrives. It is also of equal importance that the physician, upon arrival, be capable of taking over responsibility for more definitive management of the patient.

Traditionally, rural hospital emergency rooms are not staffed at all. Floor nurses "float" to the emergency room (ER) as need dictates. This technique is deficient in two ways. First and foremost is the marked variation in competence of the general nursing staff. The majority of general nurses, either in a rural or an urban area, are not trained to initiate therapy while waiting for the physician to arrive. Some nurses with intensive care unit experience have gained greater autonomy and confidence in beginning therapeutic maneuvers, usually under the general mantle of a set of prearranged standing orders.

But if there is no special in-service training, one cannot assume that all nurses called upon to take charge of an emergency have either the requisite capability or self-assurance. Second, there is always the risk, although small, that the nursing staff will be spread too thinly to attend to problems on the ward and respond to an emergency in the ER. Some system of backup is necessary to provide adequate depth of coverage in the case of simultaneous demands.

An obvious recourse is to provide systematic in-service training for rural nurses in the principles and practice of emergency care. This is an absolute necessity in those hospitals where floor nurses will be responsible for the initial hospital contact with the emergency patient. The state of Vermont has developed a 30-hour in-service training program in emergency medical care for the nurse, and this instructional package is available from the Vermont State Health Department.[26] Portions of existing EMT courses can also be adapted by local physicians and nursing directors to serve as the core of such a training module. Considering the substantial investment of people's time that is made in training the EMT-A's who ride the ambulance, an even more modest amount of time spent in nursing training can markedly improve the response capability of the entire system.

Another strategy adopted by some rural hospitals has been to utilize physician's assistants (PAs) and nurse practitioners (NPs) to staff rural emergency rooms. Many urban emergency rooms have turned to full-time physician emergency room groups that provide full-time coverage, an impractical solution for rural areas. Using PAs and NPs provides a way to insure 24-hour coverage without incurring the prohibitively high cost associated with a physician ER group. Rural physicians often favor this sort of arrangement because it relieves them of the burdensome responsibility of coming to the emergency room for the routine outpatient demands that are increasingly made upon it. In a study in a 205-bed hospital in Maryland, half of the cases in the emergency room could be handled by physician's assistants.[27] In addition, it is highly likely that in the one-third of truly urgent cases, the physician's assistant could have initiated treatment until the physician could arrive.

A more far-reaching approach to the staffing of rural emergency rooms was initiated in Virginia with the creation of a training program for emergency nurse practitioners, nurses with special postgraduate training in emergency care.[28] Sponsored by the University of Virginia, the nine-month program is split into three discontinuous time periods. Part of the training occurs at the university campus, but the majority of the training takes place in full-staffed community emergency rooms and ultimately in the home institutions of the nurses themselves. At the completion of the program, the nurses are eligible for state certification as nurse practitioners and can also be accredited as EMT-A instructors.

This ambitious program has the promise of providing targeted training to well-motivated rural nurses. The amount of commitment required by a nine-month program is probably too demanding for most rural nurses and fiscally impossible for the rural hospitals that select and sponsor the nurses for study. But if at least one nurse in each institution acquired this level of training, that individual could then translate the training into an operational plan for the rural emergency room, an ongoing in-service program, and a much improved ability to handle emergency cases.

Accompanying the heightened attention to emergency care has been the classification of hospitals according to their ability to handle emergency cases. This classification system sorts hospitals according to the types of physicians that are continuously available within the hospital walls. Hospitals with full-time emergency room staffs have a higher rating than those whose staff members are on call; teaching hospitals with residents from surgery and orthopedics, for example, receive a higher rating still. The purpose of this program is to provide automatic triage in emergency cases. Ambulance crews with a certain type of victim will automatically bypass hospitals whose classification indicates that they may be unable to care for the patient they are transporting.

Although classification does provide a certain reflex simplicity to the problem of patient destination amidst competing potential hospitals, it is not a panacea for rural hospitals. Some patients in rural areas cannot tolerate the increased transport times needed to bring them to a hospital that—by virtue of its designation as some sort of trauma center—can theoretically deal definitively with the problem with which they are presented. It is, paradoxically, those patients with the most life-threatening problems who can least afford further treatment delay. Every hospital must be able to provide the rudimentary and critical underpinnings of emergency response—

resuscitation and stabilization.[29] Only when the patient is in stable condition does the rural hospital or the EMS system have the luxury of referring the patient for more sophisticated care if indicated.

The minimum standards for a basic hospital emergency room in a rural setting follow logically from the services that the hospital must be able to deliver to support life in the face of major illness or injury. Paraphrasing Waller, these basic facilities include the following elements:

1. A two-way radio communications system linked to all ambulances in the local EMS region and to adjoining hospitals, with staff capable of operating it around the clock.

2. A trained person in the hospital at all times who can perform the rudimentary elements of resuscitation and stabilization, including airway management, identifying and managing lethal cardiac arrhythmias, control of bleeding, and acute volume replacement. This person can be a nurse, nurse practitioner, PA, or physician, but one of them must be predictably present at all times.

3. Standing orders and protocols covering the activities of the hospital personnel while the physician is en route to the hospital.

4. The hospital emergency room must be able to get a physician with adequate skills in emergency care to the hospital ER within 15 minutes. In most instances, this necessitates a voice paging system for the on-call physician.

5. Laboratory tests and x-ray films should be obtainable within 30 minutes at all times.

6. The hospital emergency room should have a standardized set of basic emergency equipment and a system for monitoring its readiness and restocking used supplies.

7. The hospital should appoint a multidisciplinary emergency department committee with a regular meeting schedule and the responsibility to audit the operation of the emergency room and recommend and implement needed improvements.

8. The emergency room should be well identified by appropriate signs and easy to find and enter in all weather conditions.

9. Protocols should be developed that indicate who can be con-

tacted when additional help is needed and where patients can be transferred when the needs arise. These protocols should be widely disseminated and regularly reviewed for their currency. It is essential that the emergency room staff be able to get help by phone at all times for all types of conditions.

10. Arrangements should be made in advance for the physical transfer of patients to other facilities. There should be appropriate mutual operating agreements with adjoining jurisdictions and formal linkages with the various centers, such as burn therapy units and neonatal intensive care units (ICUs) to which the particular rural hospital refers.

11. A simple data collection system should exist that will generate reliable information about all emergency cases cared for in the emergency room. These should include diagnostic, therapeutic, and demographic information, as well as data concerning the outcomes of the cases. These data should serve as the basis for the ongoing monitoring of the adequacy of the emergency room, comparison with other facilities with established norms, and as a basis for research.

These elements will form the foundation of a satisfactory rural hospital emergency system. More sophisticated rural emergency departments are attainable but very expensive; they depend largely on the constant in-hospital availability of physicians, either generalists or—in the more advanced facility—a variety of specialists whose talents are particularly germane to emergency work. But the emphasis in most rural communities should be on assuring the existence of the basic system. If the hospital is not able to satisfy this basic level of performance, it is a dangerous delusion for it to claim to provide emergency care. Nothing is more catastrophic than to go through the laborious and time-consuming process of getting the patient out of the ambulance and into the emergency room only to find that the staff present are unable to cope with the critical needs of the patient. It can be argued that if a rural hospital is unable to provide basic emergency care, there is little justification for its continued existence. The rural hospital is capable of fulfilling this function, but it requires recognition of the problem and a concentrated coordinated attempt to build a satisfactory emergency capability.

ORGANIZATION OF RURAL EMERGENCY SYSTEMS

The components of the rural EMS system are only as good as the organizational glue that holds them together. The EMS systems are the spokes that extend throughout the service area providing access to medical care to those patients who are most critically in need. But because it is an outreach effort depending upon the coordination of disparate groups of volunteers and professionals and the integrated working of a sometimes cantankerous collection of technological instruments, it is subject to malfunction. The organizational framework must be solid, stable, simple, and supportable, or else the fanciest gadgetry and best trained technicians will be useless.

The massive federal investment in EMS—especially when combined with state and foundation contributions—allowed a quantum jump in the overall quality of emergency medical services in the United States. However, as with many federal programs, the money was injected as a fairly discrete pulse, without much consideration and with little allowance for replacement of aging equipment or the operational costs of the system. As a result, the major impact of the legislation was to put the physical components of the system in place, raise awareness of the importance of the issue, and forge a consensus on some logical approaches to provision of this vital human service. The future viability of the system is exquisitely dependent on the ability of local areas to continue to manage and improve what they have started.

This is particularly true in rural areas. In an urban situation, it is feasible to delegate responsibility for EMS management to a component of the city or county government. Professional EMS coordinators and paid paramedics can be supported through relatively small and politically popular taxes. Rural systems do not have this luxury. First, the cost per case in the EMS system is higher in the rural areas because of increased transport distances and the large fixed costs engendered in erecting a system that will deal with relatively few cases. Second, town and county governments in rural areas do not have the resources to manage a system of this type.

The EMS systems in rural areas depend on volunteer labor. Citizens, contributing their time, comprise the ambulance corps. Health professionals volunteer their time to organize and teach EMT courses and to sit on the inevitable committees and review groups involved in making the project flow. Fortunately, emergency services assume a very high priority in the lives of rural residents, and EMS activities attract many volunteers and contributors. Yet, for the system to run smoothly, there must be a professionally organized core.

The major organizational requirement for a smoothly running rural EMS system is for a centralized focus of administrative responsibility. The logical location for that focus is the rural hospital, which is also best equipped to serve as the coordinator of emergency services from the professional as well as the managerial standpoint. Hospitals, be they public or private, are legal entities with existing boards of directors and, for the most part, nonprofit status. Some, as extensions of local government, also have taxing authority. It would appear to be in their own self-interest to promote the hospital by beefing up and receiving credit for emergency services. It also provides a mechanism for integrating the welter of personnel involved with EMS, from the EMT to the consulting physician.

A common pattern over the last decade has been for the rural hospital to assume management of the ambulance system. The Memorial Hospital in Menomonie, Wisconsin, replaced the local funeral parlor as the authority responsible for the local ambulance system in an effort that brought together the city council, hospital board, and other community leaders.[30] In Tulare County, California, the ambulance service was transferred to the hospital from the fire department, and as a result of this transition a special department was created within the hospital to deal with a range of emergency-related services.[31] Regional EMS plans, in general, use the existing hospitals as the nodes around which the system is structured.[32] It follows logically that these same focal points be identified as the administrative skeleton that keeps the individual pieces of the system from collapsing under the weight of their own complexity.

An interesting demonstration of this principle is seen in the experience of Noble County, Indiana, where the county commissioners contracted with the board of directors at the local hospital for provision of EMS services. The commissioners appropriated the funds to cover the inevitable deficit that such a system entails, and the hospital took responsibility for establishing and operating the system. An obvious advantage of this mechanism is that existing hospital resources—plant, personnel, and administration—can be tapped for the EMS system. This greatly reduces the fixed costs for both the traditional hospital functions and the EMS system, spreading underutilized resources across a broader range of responsibilities.

Another advantage of this arrangement is that rural hospitals have already developed relationships with a variety of other institutions outside their area that are also vital to a healthy rural EMS system. The same surgeon who provides consultation and backup to the rural hospital's operating room can participate in training and setting standards for the care of trauma victims. The neonatal ICU personnel to whom sick infants are transferred will also usually be willing to review protocols for emergency stabilization of children. Tertiary care cardiologists who receive referrals for patients requiring coronary angiography can also help assure that the cardiac resuscitation equipment in the emergency room is appropriate.

Moreover, rural hospitals have at least some capacity to wend their way through the maze of regulatory agencies whose rules permeate every nook of the health care industry. Although rural hospitals themselves are often at a disadvantage when dealing with remote and at times obdurate licensing agencies and third-party payers, they at least share a language in common. In addition, rural hospitals form a political constituency with considerable influence.

In summary, emergency medical services are an essential component of any rural health care system. It is an area that engages the interest, enthusiasm, and support of almost every citizen. More than almost any other realm of medicine, it breaks down the sometimes formidable barriers separating the professional from the patient. The rural emergency medical system depends on citizen participation, not only in bake sales and committee meetings, but also in providing life-saving care on a desolate road during a winter storm. The rural EMS system can provide the impetus to mobilize an entire community to improve its medical care and can be the foundation for a transformation of all aspects of the health care system.

REFERENCES

1. Perry BC, Chrisinger EW, Gordon MJ, Henze WA: A practice based study of trauma in a rural community. *Journal of Family Practice* 10(6):1039–1043, 1980.
2. Waller JA: Emergency health services in areas of low population density. *Journal of the American Medical Association* 207:2255–2258, 1969.
3. Kane R, Dean M, Solomon M: An evaluation of rural health care research. *Evaluation Quarterly* 3:139–189, 1979.
4. Smith BA: EMS communications development: History and commentary. *IEEE Transportation Vehicular Technology* VT–25:97–100, November 1976.
5. Andrews RB: Viewing EMS as a system, in NCHSR Research Proceeding Series: *Emergency Medical Services Systems as a Health Services Research Setting.* DHEW Publication No. (PHS) 79–3233, Government Printing Office, 1978.
6. Boyd DR: Emergency medical services development: A national initiative. *IEEE Transportation Vehicular Technology* VT–25(4):104–115, November 1976.
7. Haddon W: Advances in the epidemiology of injuries as a basis for public policy. *Public Health Reports* 95:411–421, 1980.
8. Haddon W: Energy damage and ten countermeasure strategies. *Journal of Trauma* 13:321–331, 1973.
9. Mayer JD: Emergency medical service: Delays, response time, and survival. *Medical Care* 17:818–827, 1979.
10. Mayer JD: Paramedic response time and survival from cardiac arrest. *Social Science and Medicine* 13D:267–271, 1979.
11. Frazier WH, Cannon JF: Emergency medical technician performance evaluation, in NCHSR *Research Report Series.* DHEW Publication No. (PHS) 78–3211, Government Printing Office, May 1978.
12. Spoor JE: Rural advanced EMT training. *Emergency Medical Service* 6:77–78, September–October 1977.
13. Waller JA, Gettinger CE: Rural emergency medical services. *EMT Journal* 1:31–35, 1977.
14. Thays JA: Some innovative approaches to providing emergency services in a rural area. *EMT Journal* 1:36–37, 1977.
15. Volz RA: Optimum ambulance location in semi-rural areas. *Transportation Science* 5:193–203. 1971.
16. Jarvis JP, Stevenson KA, Willemain TR: *A Simple Procedure for the Allocation of Ambulances in Semi-Rural Areas.* Technical Report No. TR–13–75, Operations Research Center. Cambridge, Massachusetts Institute of Technology, 1975.

17. Daberkow SG: Location and cost of ambulances serving a rural area. *Health Services Research* 12:299–311, 1977.
18. Doeksen GA, Frye J, Green BL: *Economics of rural ambulance service in the Great Plains.* Agricultural Economics Report No. 308, Economic Research Service. United States Department of Agriculture, 1975.
19. Proctor HJ, Acai SA: Assets and liabilities of helicopter evacuation in support of emergency medical services. *Journal of the American College of Emergency Physicians* 4:543–547, 1975.
20. *Helicopters in emergency medical service: NHTSA experience to date,* in US Department of Transportation, National Highway Traffic Safety Administration Stock No. 5003–00112. US Government Printing Office, 1972.
21. Jordan RF, Wegmann FJ, Carter EC: *Planning a helicopter transportation system to augment emergency and regional medical programs in a test region of West Virginia.* Document No. PB 195 801. Springfield, Virginia, National Technical Information Service.
22. Cowley RA, Hudson F, Scanlon E, et al: An economical and proved helicopter program for transporting the critically ill and injured patient in Maryland. *Journal of Trauma* 13:1029–1038, 1973.
23. Henry WJ: Alternative to 911. *Emergency Medicine Today* 3(9):1–4, September 1974.
24. Penterman DG: A case study in telecommunications. *Emergency Medical Service* 3(3):16, 1974.
25. Waller JA: Categorizing hospital emergency departments in rural areas. *Clinical Medicine* 82:41–47, 1975.
26. Weiner MA, Gettinger CE, Waller JA, et al: Inservice training for rural nurses in emergency care concepts and skills. *Journal of Emergency Nursing* 1:16–23, March–April 1975.
27. Golomb HM, Herrold SR: An alternative staffing proposal for emergency rooms: Three year experience in a rural hospital. *Journal of the American Medical Association* 228:329–331, 1974.
28. Geolot D, Alongi S, Edlich RF: Emergency nurse practitioners: An answer to an emergency case crisis in rural hospitals. *JACEP* 6:355–357, 1977.
29. Waller JA: A rural EMS categorization system. *Journal of the American Hospital Association* 49:111–116, 1974.
30. Jensen KE: A hospital-based ambulance service. *Hospitals* 46:65–69, 1972.
31. McClendon EL, Fikes JM: Rural ambulance service. *Hospitals* 45:68–71, 1971.
32. Doeksen GA, Anderson LG, Whitlow WM: *A community development guide for emergency medical services.* Oklahoma Department of Transportation, 1978.

CHAPTER 6

The Rural Hospital: Problems and Prospects

The rural hospital is the center of the rural health care system. The rural hospital plays a significant role in the community of which it is a part—functionally, symbolically, and economically. A rural community will fight to save its hospital even when it has lost its last apparent vestige of utility; the hospital ranks with the church and the school as one of those elements of rural society through which communities define themselves.

In Chapters 4 and 5, we discussed the means by which rural communities maintain their capacity to provide basic primary and emergency medical care. In much the same way that the physician is the central figure in providing medical care, the hospital is the institution around which medical care is oriented. There is a symbiotic relationship between the physician and the hospital, a relationship that is much more intimate in rural areas, where physicians are few and hospitals are small.[1] The relationship between the rural physician and the hospital is more characteristic of a small family than of an impersonal bureaucracy. Without hospitals, physicians are reluctant to come to or stay in rural communities, and without physicians, hospitals cannot remain financially solvent.[2-4]

The rural hospital is fundamental to the physician in several ways. As discussed in Chapter 4, it acts as a workshop for that portion of the physician's medical activities that require large amounts of capital investment and labor-intensive care. This tends to reduce the financial risks the physician must take to start and maintain a practice, since the costs of supporting the hospital are borne by the hospital and the community itself, not the physician. This allows physicians to generate more total income by increasing the spectrum of services that they have to offer while decreasing the amount of money they must invest in expensive, infrequently used, and rapidly outdated technology.

Perhaps more important from the community perspective is the hospital's contribution to maintenance of standards of care, what Somers calls the "principal center for development of quality measurements and control."[5] Although a relatively small proportion of all ambulatory patients are hospitalized, they are that fraction of the population requiring the most intense concentration of services.[6] Physicians and hospital personnel make decisions in the hospital that often have life-or-death implications for the patients for whom they are responsible. It is in the hospital where the physician receives the informal and structured scrutiny of peers, where frequently new methods and techniques first appear, and where the bulk of continuing education is transmitted. The physician without a hospital practice is in danger of obsolescence, and it is no accident that inadequate physicians sometimes choose to settle in small rural communities that lack hospitals.

Hospitals can also be the conduit for change in the community.[7,8] Rural hospitals can help translate the aspirations of the community into new types of services for the rural area. Hospital boards, be they government or private nonprofit, often serve as the applicant agency for state or federal grants to improve the health care delivery system. Although it is common for rural hospitals to display a certain inherent conservatism, their existence in the community provides an operational base from which innovation can proceed.

The explicit task of the rural hospital is to provide inpatient services. There is little agreement as to which specific services should be available. A major question in the current debate surrounding rural hospitals is the degree to which regionalization and centralization of services should be mandated. During the last decade rural hospitals have been pressured to constrict the scope of services they offer patients and to decrease the size of their operations or close altogether. In an attempt to gain control over the escalating costs of health care—the greatest part of which is directly attributable to hospital care—planners and regulators have attempted to curtail hospital expansion and pare "excess" beds. By the same token, planners have invoked quality considerations in addition to economics to argue that small rural hospitals provide inferior care in areas like obstetrics because of inadequate volume, obsolete equipment, and poorly trained personnel.

Rural hospitals find themselves in a quandary. On the one hand, they appear to be fundamental to the capacity of a rural community to retain and expand basic health services. On the other hand, powerful external forces threaten their financial and professional equilibrium, and the quality and appropriateness of the care they do provide is brought into question. In this chapter, we will review these issues in an attempt to define the role that a rural hospital can play within the larger health care system, maintaining adequate quality of care and financial stability while providing basic services to the rural population. In the final analysis, there is no unitary formula that can be applied to all situations, but it is possible to identify those characteristics of a rural hospital that are most vital to its success in the broader sense of that term.

We first will review the statistics that illustrate the place of the rural hospital within the context of the American hospital industry. We then discuss the internal operating characteristics of the rural hospital, using an economic model as a framework for the discussion. This discussion is followed by a review of some of the environmental factors that impinge on the rural hospital, such as planning and regulation, and the somewhat paradoxical nature of the market for hospital services, which prompts external attempts at regulation. We conclude with a review of some of the options available to the rural hospital to assist it in both meeting its objectives of service to the community and ensuring its economic survival.

THE RURAL HOSPITAL IN A NATIONAL PERSPECTIVE

Rural hospitals comprise a significant proportion of all United States hospitals. Table 6.1 illustrates the relative importance of the rural hospital in the national health care system. Half of all hospitals

TABLE 6.1. U.S. Community Hospital Characteristics by Location, 1979

	Nonmetropolitan	Percent of U.S. Total	Metropolitan	Percent of U.S. Total
Number of hospitals	2,886	49.4	2,956	50.6
Number of beds	249,350	25.3	734,344	74.7
Average bed size	86		248	
Admissions	8,768,109	25.0	26,331,122	75.0
Occupancy (%)	66.7		76.4	
Surgical operations	3,615,141	19.8	14,653,440	80.2
Births	799,648	24.3	2,487,364	75.7
Total expenses per bed	43,829		74,999	

Source: *Hospital Statistics, 1980 Edition*, American Hospital Association, Chicago, Illinois.

are outside of standard metropolitan statistical areas (SMSAs). These hospitals have certain characteristics that distinguish them from their urban counterparts. They are on the average one-third as big as urban hospitals, have predictably lower occupancy rates, and provide roughly one-quarter of inpatient services in obstetrics, surgery, and general medical services.

Rural hospitals are considerably less capitalized than are urban hospitals, both for the institutions as a whole and when computed on a per-bed basis. By the same token, rural hospitals are less costly to operate, with the cost per bed 58 percent of that prevailing in urban areas.

Tables 6.2 through 6.4 provide some additional insight into the characteristics of rural hospitals. Although these data are classified by hospital size rather than location, the majority of hospitals of fewer than 100 beds are in rural areas, and the smaller the hospital, the more likely it is to be in a rural community. Examining the characteristics of hospitals as a function of their size allows us to gain additional information about smaller and rural hospitals.

Table 6.2 reveals that hospitals of fewer than 100 beds comprise approximately one-half of all hospitals in the United States, essentially identical with the relative proportion of hospitals located in nonmetropolitan areas. Small hospitals, when considered as a class, assume less importance than do rural hospitals when examined with respect to the total amount of health services produced. While rural hospitals account for one-quarter of the beds and almost one-quarter of the various hospital services, small hospitals as a class have only about 15 percent of the total beds and an even smaller proportion of the total services. One must conclude that although most rural hospitals are small and most small hospitals are rural, there are exceptions to both of these rules.

Table 6.3 shows that small hospitals differ from larger institutions in their ownership patterns. Where the predominant mode of ownership in the country at large is that of the nongovernment, nonprofit hospital, a disproportionately large percentage of rural hospitals are owned by local governments. This is a reflection of the role that rural hospitals play as a part of community life; they are seen as an extension of the public responsibilities of local and county government, a necessary service akin to schools or police. This also stems from the somewhat more unstable financial characteristics of

TABLE 6.2. U.S. Short-Term General Hospital Characteristics by Hospital Size, 1979

Hospital Size	Number of Hospitals	Percent of Total	Number of Beds	Percent of Total	Number of Admissions	Percent of Total	Number of Surgical Operations	Percent of Total
6–24	310	5.1	5,917	0.6	189,178	0.5	50,927	0.3
25–49	1,121	18.3	40,579	3.8	1,345,092	3.7	368,477	2.0
50–99	1,459	23.9	104,677	9.9	3,631,500	9.9	1,380,556	7.3
≥ 100	3,219	52.7	909,155	85.7	31,474,310	85.9	16,967,765	90.4
Total	6,109	100.0	1,060,368	100.0	36,640,080	100.0	18,767,725	100.0

Source: *Hospital Statistics, 1980 Edition,* American Hospital Association, Chicago, Illinois.

TABLE 6.3. Control Characteristics of U.S. Short-Term General Hospitals by Hospital Size, 1979

Hospital Size	Nongovernment Not for Profit		Investor Owned for Profit		Local Government		State Government		Federal Government		Total Number of Hospitals
	No.	Percent of All Hospitals of this Size	No.	Percent of All Hospitals of this Size	No.	Percent of All Hospitals of this Size	No.	Percent of All Hospitals of this Size	No.	Percent of All Hospitals of this Size	
6–24	88	28.4	40	12.9	133	42.9	13	4.2	36	11.6	310
25–49	389	34.7	130	11.6	505	45.0	32	2.8	65	5.8	1,121
50–99	658	58.6	183	16.3	563	50.2	20	1.8	35	3.1	1,459
≥ 100	2,128	66.1	342	10.6	494	15.3	69	2.2	186	5.8	3,219
Total	3,263	53.4	695	11.4	1,695	27.7	134	2.2	322	5.3	6,109

Source: *Hospital Statistics, 1980 Edition*, American Hospital Association, Chicago, Illinois.

TABLE 6.4. Distribution of Community Hospitals by Bed-Size Category, 1969 and 1979

Bed Size	Number of Hospitals		Percent Change
	1969	1979	
6–24	423	269	−36.4
25–49	1,365	1,055	−22.7
50–99	1,485	1,448	− 2.5
100–199	1,264	1,378	+ 9.0
200–299	572	718	+25.5
300–399	339	401	+18.3
400–499	194	251	+29.4
500 or more	211	322	+52.6
Totals	5,853	5,842	

Source: *Hospital Statistics, 1980 Edition*, American Hospital Association, Chicago, Illinois.

rural hospitals, such that creation of a public entity with taxing and bonding authority is the only way many rural hospitals maintain their solvency.

Table 6.4 provides some sobering insight into the relative health of the small and rural hospital. In the decade from 1969 to 1979, although the number of hospitals in the country decreased less than one percent, there was a profound shift in their distribution by size. Hospitals with fewer than 100 beds became a much smaller proportion of the total hospital scene, while larger hospitals became more prevalent. While exact data are lacking, undoubtedly the changes are due to two separate but complementary causes. Hospitals tended to add beds during this period across the entire size spectrum, and many small hospitals closed. Since the smallest hospitals are those most likely to be in rural areas, and since they suffered the most profound attrition in their numbers, it is likely that many rural communities are today without the hospitals that they had a decade earlier.

We can conclude that the rural hospital remains an important component of the health care scene but that its future is troubled. In the following section we will review some of the factors that are contributing to the malaise of and the stress upon the rural hospital.

INTERNAL OPERATING CHARACTERISTICS OF THE RURAL HOSPITAL—AN ECONOMIC APPROACH

Hospitals have become the core of the health care delivery system. Hospitals are the focus of the dramatic and the costly; they have become by far the largest single component of the health care budget, and their relative and absolute importance continues to increase. Hospital costs have risen at a rate much higher than inflation, and the proliferation of new technologies and new personnel needed to operate them shows no sign of abating.

The rapidly rising cost of health care has become a fiscal obsession with government at all levels; particularly in an era of sluggish overall financial growth, the increased diversion of public monies to finance health services limits government flexibility in all other areas. The result has been a multifaceted, and so far largely unsuccessful, attempt to restrain rising costs, with the thrust of cost containment logically directed first and foremost at the hospital industry.

Rural hospitals as a class are subject to the same pressures applied to the hospital industry in general. Because of their small size and limited administrative capability, they have more difficulty complying with regulations and devising the effective organizational strategies that allow larger hospitals to maintain their autonomy. In addition to the heightened impact of regulation on rural hospitals, these institutions face a set of problems that are unique to their situation.

To understand the very real threats to the continued existence of rural hospitals, it is essential to understand how hospitals work as economic organisms and what the major issues are that confront hospitals in general. Hospitals are at the same time complex, multiproduct firms and altruistic social service organizations. To understand rural hospitals, we need to delve into the economic life of hospitals and the relationship of fiscal concerns to the type and quality of care that hospitals produce.

Hospitals differ significantly one from the other. They differ in size, in the services they offer, in the complexity and type of patients for whom they care. In many ways, hospitals are akin to clothing factories. Although each factory makes apparel designed to be worn, there is immense variation in the cost, shape, elegance, quality, and purpose of each piece of clothing. In the same way, the factories that make different kinds of clothes vary in the skill of the personnel they hire, the sophistication of the machines they use, the types of materials they purchase, and the way in which they are organized. This combination of ingredients that the factory uses to produce its product is called the *production function*, and in order to analyze and compare hospitals we must understand their production functions as well.

One way to understand the hospital's production function is to look at those factors that affect the average cost to the hospital of producing hospital services. This method is useful because costs vary dramatically among hospitals, and rapidly rising costs have led to the application of regulatory controls designed to bring the health care budget under control. Economists have represented hospital cost functions as follows:

$$AC = f(O, M, Q, P, E)$$

where average cost (AC) is a function of the variables O, M, Q, P, and E. O stands for hospital output, M is the product mix or complexity of the services provided, Q is quality, P is the price of the goods and services hospitals use to keep running, and E is efficiency.[9] Although this equation is somewhat oversimplified in that it ignores certain additional variables, analyzing each of these elements in turn will allow us to understand the internal operating characteristics of rural hospitals and review what is known about the effects of rural location on each of these characteristics.

Before considering the way in which these variables interact to determine the final cost of hospital services, we must realize that we usually are forced to deal only with direct, measurable prices that hospitals charge for their services. The true cost of hospitalization is significantly greater than the charge that the hospital makes and includes both indirect costs and externalities. The major indirect cost is travel, the amount of money expended by patients, patients' families, and hospital staff to get to the hospital. This is obviously a critical element in the placement of rural hospitals; the nearer the hospital to the center of its service area, the lower the total travel costs. In addition to travel costs, which are actual out-of-packet costs and can be measured, there are external costs that are less quantifiable. An example of an external cost is the degree to which the absence of a hospital makes the town unattractive to potential new businesses. There is a real economic cost involved, but it may be very difficult to calculate.

HOSPITAL OUTPUT—ECONOMIES OF SCALE AND THE HOSPITAL INDUSTRY

Many enterprises demonstrate economies of scale; as their size increases, it costs less to produce a given item. Economists have attempted to determine whether such a relationship exists in the hospital industry. The evidence is conflicting and inconclusive, but it appears that economies of scale with regard to *direct* costs exist—up to a point. Small hospitals and large hospitals appear to be more costly than medium-sized hospitals, with the lowest-cost hospital size being about 200 beds. [9-11] Figure 6.1 shows the relationship that describes this observation.

This curve, however, is flawed by the omission of the impact of travel costs on the total equation. As Berry points out, "albeit hospital services are produced subject to economies of scale, the absolute and relative magnitudes of the potential savings do not provide much of an incentive for exploitation. In fact, these cost estimates are in terms of internal monetary costs and take no account

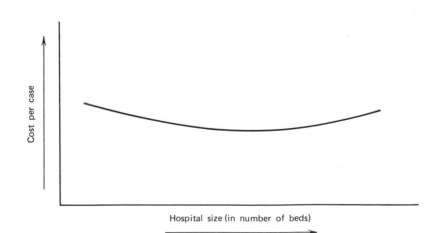

Figure 6.1. The effect of hospital size on hospital costs.

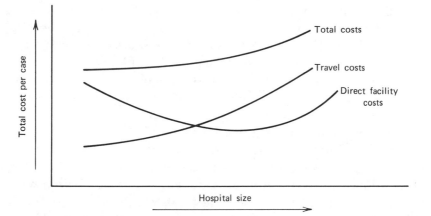

Figure 6.2. The effect of travel costs and hospital size on the cost of hospital care.

of travel costs or the costs associated with inconvenience to patients, attending physicians, or visitors. Since travel costs and inconvenience would necessarily increase if hospitals were larger and consequently served larger catchment areas, it would seem that the relative insignificance of the magnitude of economies of scale may explain the large number of relatively small hospitals."[9]

It is impossible to draw an accurate cost curve that takes into account travel costs because of the lack of reliable data. In one study the costs were substantial.[10] Patient travel accounted for only 5.9 percent of the total miles involved in hospitalization; most of the cost was sustained by hospital employees and visitors. Figure 6.2 is a hypothetical depiction of the relationship of hospital size to cost with the addition of travel costs to the equation. Although we lack the data to substantiate the upward sloping nature of the hospital cost curve, it seems plausible. No matter what the exact relationship, it seems safe to conclude that size alone is not the major determinant of the cost of care of any given hospital.

COMPLEXITY AND COST

Hospitals differ greatly in what they do and who they serve. The range of services a hospital is prepared to offer is known as the *scope of service*; the proportion of patients with various illnesses that the hospital actually serves is known as the *case mix.* The scope of services and the case mix are not necessarily well matched; hospitals may "gear up" to provide fairly sophisticated services but may have a patient clientele whose range of medical problems rarely require them. These two aspects of complexity of the product the hospital provides turn out to explain most of the observed disparity in cost among different hospitals.

There is some evidence that hospitals go through a predictable pattern of evolution, adding additional services in a set and reproducible way.[12] Hospitals begin as basic service institutions, offering the traditional obstetric, surgical, and medical services, with few embellishments. In the next phase hospitals go through a period of quality enhancement, improving the depth with which they can handle the basic services they are providing but without changing the actual scope of services. In the third stage they add more complex medical services, expanding their scope of services. In their final stage they become full-scale community medical centers, providing not only direct inpatient services, but also outreach and support services, and also take on certain educational functions.[9,13]

The impact of a hospital's scope of service per se on cost is controversial. Berry was able to use standard lists of hospital services to distinguish among eight fairly cohesive groups of hospitals based on their relative scope of services and to show that this classification had an impact on cost.[14] Edwards and her associates were able to use a scaling technique to array hospitals along a spectrum from least to most complex with regard to scope of services; although this explained most of the observed variance in costs, the majority of the hospitals were clustered at the lower end of their scale, and it was difficult to separate them.[12] Klastorin and Watts have worked on techniques to cluster hospitals into homogeneous groups based on internal operating characteristics in order to formulate rational prospective reimbursement schemes.[15,16] When they used scope of service as a surrogate for case mix, they found that they were unable to explain the majority of the observed variance in cost.

Many observers have been very critical of the scope of service approach to distinguishing among hospitals and the methodological techniques used to measure them.[17] In general, direct or indirect measures of case mix have been sought as a better way to compare hospitals. Various measures have emerged, and researchers have applied them to a variety of data bases. Lave and Lave looked at the composition of cases by using diagnostic codes, as well as the complexity of therapy used as a measure of case mix.[18] Schumacher and his collaborators used the degree to which a service was centralized as a proxy for case mix complexity.[19] In this technique, diagnoses that tended to be concentrated in large tertiary centers were judged to be more complex than diagnoses that were spread among all the hospitals in the state. Zaretsky constructed a spectrum of case mix complexity from hospital discharge summaries and formulated a scope of service index using the previously mentioned scaling techniques.[13] Applying this model to a sample of California hospitals explained 69 percent of the observed cost variation. The author concludes that "the cost function estimates described above suggest that when adjustments are made for service mix and case mix, size or volume does not greatly influence the cost per case."

What emerges from a review of the many studies relating hospital complexity to cost is that both the scope of services and the case mix are extremely important characteristics of hospitals and are the primary source of differences in cost among hospitals. Whether hospital costs depend more on what hospitals "gear up" to do than on what they actually end up doing, or whether case mix is the most direct measure of the hospital's primary output, both factors must be considered in analyzing hospital performance.[9,16]

Rural hospitals do not fit into the prevailing pattern with regard to complexity of cases treated. Rural hospitals tend to treat more complex cases than do urban hospitals of comparable size. In the Maryland study by Schumacher previously cited, there were marked differences between hospitals in standard metropolitan statistical areas (SMSAs) and non-SMSAs.[19] Rural hospitals were found to have a significantly higher proportion of cases with high clinical complexity. A similar pattern was observed by Lave in Pennsylvania; again, rural hospitals were found to care for a more complex spectrum of patients than small urban hospitals. Lave speculates that "the general tendency of small urban hospitals to produce medical care that is less complex than that of small rural hospitals may be related to the fact that the ratio of hospital beds to population is much higher [in urban areas]."[18] However, a better explanation may be that rural hospitals are more likely to treat all segments of the population than are small urban hospitals and must be prepared to manage complex clinical problems that, in an urban area, would be quickly referred to larger institutions.

It is clear that, on the basis of the complexity variable, rural hospitals might be expected to be more costly than urban hospitals and should be reimbursed commensurately. This has been specifically recognized in certain cases in which prospective reimbursement schemes have been proposed. Some forms of prospective reimbursement try to restrain costs by paying hospitals on the basis of what they propose to do instead of what it costs them after the fact. Since case mix and scope of service account for the majority of the variation in cost among hospitals, an effective prospective reimbursement plan depends on the ability to group similar hospitals into categories that are internally homogeneous with regard to the complexity of the patients they treat. In order to take into account the special characteristics of rural hospitals, it is necessary to treat them differently and reimburse them more generously than urban hospitals of similar size and scope. This is explicitly recognized by Klastorin et al. in their work on prospective reimbursement: "Hospital costs will also be higher in rural areas where demand is not sufficient to extensively utilize indivisible pieces of hospital capital. Higher prices to cover higher costs would be sustained in the market since, for some set of basic services, it is less costly to support an underutilized facility than travel where services can be obtained or to do without."[15]

In summary, we see that clinical complexity and intensity, not hospital size, account for most of the large variation in hospital costs. Rural hospitals, because they function as unique community institutions, tend to treat somewhat more complex patients than do urban hospitals of similar size. When travel costs are considered, the weight of evidence points to the fact that it is more economical in some cases to maintain decentralized rural hospitals than to direct patients to larger, but more remote, regional or urban facilities. However, before concluding that it is desirable to retain our current rural hospital network, we must examine the evidence that relates hospital size and location to the quality of care produced.

THE RELATIONSHIP OF HOSPITAL SIZE AND LOCATION TO QUALITY OF CARE

Quality of care is of central importance to our consideration of the status of the rural hospital. One critical observer has commented,

"The quality of services delivered in or by small community hospitals of less than 25 beds are barely tolerable from the perspective of the public interest."[20] Rural hospitals may be a vital social and economic part of rural society, but if they involve more risk for the patients who use them, it becomes difficult to justify their continued existence.

Quality is an imprecise concept; it can be applied to the mortality experienced after surgical procedures or to the taste of hospital meals. For the most part, the relatively scant information that does exist about the quality of hospital care uses mortality rates as a measure of outcome. Mortality has the advantage of being easily defined, widely recorded, and unambiguous. It has the methodological disadvantage of being relatively infrequent. Studies comparing relative mortalities are further clouded by differences in case mix, in patient sociodemographic characteristics, and by the fact that sometimes it is impossible to find out about a death resulting from a given hospitalization if the patient dies at home, in a nursing home, or at another hospital.

Despite these limitations, some provocative data exist. Roemer was one of the first researchers to examine issues of quality, using data from the governmentally supported health care system in Saskatchewan.[21] He compared the mortality rates for five major surgical procedures performed in hospitals of varying size. He found that for appendectomies, cholecystectomies, and prostatectomies, the outcome was better when the surgery was performed in a larger, more centralized hospital. The outcome of hysterectomies and herniorraphies did not vary with the location or size of the hospital. Although the study is limited by its design because patients were not well matched for demographic and clinical characteristics, this and similar studies helped to initiate interest in the process of regionalization of certain surgical services.

In a study of the medical appropriateness of hospitalization in Michigan, Riedel and Fitzpatrick used hospital discharge data to examine a number of common medical diagnoses.[22] The criteria used to measure appropriateness were formulated by panels of medical experts. For patients with common diagnoses, only two groups—those with diabetes and urinary tract infections—were unnecessarily hospitalized according to the criteria. With regard to urinary tract infections, smaller hospitals showed a higher rate of inappropriate admissions. However, this observation was accounted for entirely by small urban hospitals, and the smaller rural hospitals actually had fewer unnecessary admissions for this illness. An additional important factor was the source of payment. Insured patients were more likely to be inappropriately hospitalized. With regard to physician training, specialists had fewer inappropriate admissions than generalists for urinary tract infections, but a greater proportion in the case of diabetes.

A major wave of controversy was generated in the late 1960s by the findings of the National Halothane Study.[23] Set up to examine the safety of the commonly used anaesthetic gas halothane, the study team unexpectedly observed that in the sample of hospitals that were studied there was a 24-fold variation in the surgical mortality rate, varying from 0.1 to 3.0 percent of all surgical cases. After the age, sex, and clinical condition of the patient, the type of operation, and the year in which it was performed were adjusted for, a tenfold difference remained. Although the study team was unable to explain the observed difference or relate it to size or location of hospitals, their findings indicated for the first time that there was considerable variability in the quality of care provided by American hospitals.

A similar set of studies completed in England has also shown variations in surgical mortality rates. In 1971, a group of British investigators took one operation, prostatectomies, and compared the outcome between teaching hospitals and smaller community hospitals.[24] Again, the authors observed the same differences that Roemer had noted in Saskatchewan—regional hospitals had a significantly higher mortality rate. However, the authors went a step further and analyzed the actual case records involved. The difference in observed mortality turned out to be attributable to the class of patients involved; community hospitals dealt with a group of very sick emergency patients whom teaching hospitals never saw, and the difference in outcome could be explained by this disparity. The actual mortality rates for matched patients was identical.

The most recent study of this relationship was reported by Luft and coworkers and grew out of the observed discrepancies in the National Halothane Study.[25] Using a national sample of hospitals, Luft and coworkers examined mortality rates for 12 common surgical procedures in the 1,498 hospitals in their sample. Differences in the clinical severity of patients' problems were controlled by including the age and sex of patients, as well as the number of diagnoses that were recorded for each patient.

The findings were clear; for the majority of the operations studied there was a definite and reproducible relationship between the volume of procedures done and the mortality rate observed. Hospitals doing more of certain procedures had lower mortality rates.

Closer analysis of the data showed that there were three different patterns linking the volume of operations to the mortality rate. In the first group of diagnoses, the surgical outcome improved as the number of procedures increased. There were no threshold effects. This group included open-heart surgery, coronary bypass surgery, and transurethral resection of the prostate. The second group showed a volume effect; there were very clear threshold volumes beyond which doing more procedures had little or no additional impact on reducing mortality. This was the largest group and included colectomy, hip replacements, biliary tract surgery, vagotomy and pyloroplasty, and several other procedures. The third group showed essentially no impact of volume on mortality. Every hospital doing cholecystectomies had essentially the same mortality rate, and increased surgical volume did not affect the outcome.

These three curves are depicted in a simplified form in Figure 6.3. The implications for rural health planning and regionalization of surgical procedures are profound, and they are discussed more fully in Chapter 8. However, it is important to note that the authors

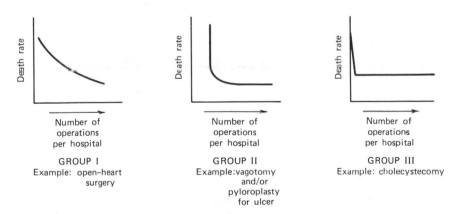

GROUP I
Example: open-heart
surgery

GROUP II
Example:vagotomy
and/or
pyloroplasty
for ulcer

GROUP III
Example: cholecystecomy

Figure 6.3. The relationship between the volume of surgical procedures and their outcome. (Luft HS, Bunker JP, Enthoven AC: Should operations be regionalized? The empirical relation between surgical volume and mortality. NEJM 301:1366, 1979.)

examine a number of other hospital characteristics—including SMSA versus non-SMSA location, the size of the hospital, and the cost of the hospital—and found that none of these variables affected the observed relationship between mortality and volume. It appears that many of the observations of earlier researchers can be explained on the basis of this apparent "institutional learning curve" and that rural location per se has little or no impact on the quality of surgical procedures measured by this technique.

Although far reaching, this study is not definitive. It does not explain which aspect of hospital function is so exquisitely volume sensitive—is it the hospital administration, the operating room team, the surgeon, or some combination of factors? Secondly, the study inadequately controls for the likelihood that some of the hospitals doing fewer procedures may be forced to operate on an emergency basis on sicker patients. The control mechanism used in this study does not account for this difference and, in fact, suggests that smaller hospitals deal with a riskier class of patients. It is interesting to note that Luft and his coworkers found prostatectomies to be one procedure that was very volume sensitive, yet the procedure is by no means as surgically delicate or complex as open-heart surgery, which fell in the same group. It may be that the explanation offered by the English investigators in their study of prostatectomy applies also in the United States.

A similar threshold effect has been observed for coronary care units, which represent the application of nonsurgical technology in the treatment of a common life-threatening disease. In a study of mostly rural community hospitals in Michigan, Stroll and coworkers observed a very marked volume effect.[26] Hospitals admitting more than 60 patients per year with myocardial infarctions—heart attacks —experience roughly half the mortality rate of hospitals admitting fewer patients: 10.9 percent versus 20.9 percent. Although the study lacks the methodologic precision of the Luft study, the result is so clear cut that it remains compelling. The data fall within the group of diagnoses depicted in group II on Figure 6.3, and it is likely that many other discrete procedures or therapeutic regimens will follow the same pattern.

Although the studies here concentrate on only a few aspects of hospital care, the combined observations are convincing. Rural hospitals are neither intrinsically better nor worse than urban hospitals.

Individual diagnoses and procedures vary greatly in their severity and their complexity, and it is likely that the curves in Figure 6.3 can be extrapolated to almost any service hospitals provide. The key to whether a given rural hospital is able to provide a certain service with an acceptable level of quality will depend on its ability to amass adequate experience in its provision. It makes no sense for rural hospitals to perform heart surgery. By the same token, it makes no sense to refer cholecystectomy patients if the operation can be done with equivalent quality in the rural hospital.

The impact of quality of care on the hospital cost function remains somewhat obscure. It is evident that increasing the intensity and range of services provided to a given homogeneous set of patients increases the cost of that care. Recent evidence supports the conclusion that, after controlling for case mix, patient outcomes are improved in hospitals with greater intensity and a shorter duration of services.[27] However, one cannot therefore conclude that quality enhancing services are economically justified in all cases. There must remain some level where the economic trade-off between increased quality and increased cost becomes prohibitive.

Moreover, outcome in the previously cited studies is measured by mortality rates. Survival and death have the advantage of being quantifiable and distinguishable events, but they may in fact not reflect the quality of the outcome for the individual patient and the patient's family. Maintaining "life" in the severely injured patient who requires complex, prolonged nursing care but does not have the ability to enjoy his or her existence may be a hollow technical triumph. We have increasingly gained the capacity to maintain a semblance of bodily function in patients beyond the time when such heroic efforts are justified. We should maintain a healthy skepticism about the incorporation of new technology into hospital care, and the ultimate resolution of some of the issues concerning quality of care awaits better end points than mortality alone.

THE RELATION OF FACTOR PRICE AND EFFICIENCY TO HOSPITAL COST

Another important reason that hospitals vary widely in their cost of care is the difference in what economists call *factor prices*; the things that hospitals need to produce hospital care, both materials and personnel, cost differing amounts in different areas. The major variation occurs in the wage rate, and Berry found that variation in wage rates was consistently significant in explaining differences in costs among hospitals.[9] This has obvious implications for rural hospitals, where wages tend to be lower, and it means that they can produce equivalent services for lower costs, all other things being equal. The importance of this difference might decrease or increase, depending on changes in the labor market. Urban unionization might increase the disparity in wage rates between rural and urban areas. On the other hand, rural areas might find that they have to offer higher salaries for certain categories of personnel to attract them to sparsely settled areas.

Efficiency reflects the ability of hospitals to meld together all the various resources that they use to provide the desired services in the most parsimonious way. Theoretically, if all other factors are controlled, any differences in cost that remain are attributable to the differences in efficiency between institutions. This is the underlying rationale for the prospective reimbursement strategy. Clustering hospitals into similar groups and then setting a reimbursement rate that is fixed will give hospitals an incentive to improve their efficiency in order to match their costs with their reimbursement level.

No clear patterns emerge with respect to the organizational status of hospitals and their relative efficiency. The only variable Berry identified that improved efficiency was having a physician as administrator. Since physicians control the expenditure of resources by the way in which they order tests and treatments, a physician administrator may have both medical insight and credibility as a colleague to assist in encouraging restraint.

It is likely that other administrative aspects also have an impact on efficiency; for example, shared purchasing should decrease costs. We will discuss various forms of shared services later in this chapter. The increasing popularity of this approach among nonprofit and for-profit hospitals suggests that sharing services does convey an advantage in terms of operational efficiency.

In summary, hospitals can be analyzed as if they were complex factories producing a variety of different products. When the economic status of a hospital is analyzed in this fashion, most of the variation in the cost of hospital services is explained by the difference in the range of services hospitals provide and the severity of the illnesses of the patients they treat. The size of the hospital is relatively unimportant. Improving the quality of the product appears to increase costs, although it is not clear by what amount. The quality with which a hospital provides a given service appears to be extremely sensitive to size, and for most services there appears to be a threshold volume, a critical mass of events, that must occur within a given time period if the hospital is to attain clinical proficiency. The costs of wages is an important component of hospital costs but is beyond the control of most hospitals.

Applying these considerations to rural hospitals yields some very useful insights. Rurality per se has almost nothing to do with whether or not hospitals are cost effective or efficient. Indeed, in an era in which travel costs are rising exponentially, it is highly likely that closing rural hospitals and centralizing hospital services will increase aggregate hospital costs. The size of the hospital operation *is* critical, not because smaller hospitals are more costly, but because the quality of care deteriorates if the volume of care is inadequate. Knowledge of the relationship between volume and quality should allow the rural hospital to select those procedures that it can perform with adequate quality simply by determining the demand for those services within its catchment area. If the demand for the procedure does not yield a volume high enough to maintain adequate quality of care, then the procedure in question should not be done within the rural hospital. On the other hand, if local demand would allow the hospital to perform the procedure with adequate quality, and if the procedure does not involve greatly added cost, then attempts should be made to incorporate that service into the rural hospital's repertoire. Neither size nor rurality per se constitutes an absolute barrier to the existence of efficient and effective rural hospitals, but careful planning is required to insure that the mix of services offered is appropriate to the population served.

THE IMPACT OF ENVIRONMENTAL FACTORS ON THE BEHAVIOR OF THE RURAL HOSPITAL

Rural hospitals do not exist in a vacuum. They are extremely sensitive not only to the local need and demand for health services, but also to the structure and function of the larger health care system. Rural hospitals do not of themselves determine what services they provide or how they will provide them; they do not have autonomy in selecting the type and number of health personnel they will employ, the size and sophistication of their plant, or the medical treatments they will offer. Advances in our understanding of disease, changes in the way physicians and nurses are trained, and technological innovations that change the norm for the way in which certain problems are approached all set the boundary conditions within which rural hospitals must operate. Society adds another layer of constraint by erecting complex health planning laws at the federal and state level, and through the creation of a regulatory framework. Together these elements further determine the environment within which rural hospitals are challenged to set logical goals for their structure and function.

Hospitals are subject to more intense external scrutiny than most other community institutions. Almost every aspect of their structure and function—from the size of the bathrooms to the quality of the food—are inspected, certified, or regulated. In addition, changes in the technology of medical care or the education of health professionals have a direct effect on the way that hospitals operate by setting the standards for treatment and determining the type and quantity of available personnel. Rural hospitals, by virtue of their small size and remoteness, have limited ability to influence these external forces with which they must contend.

A major reason that society attempts to control the activities of hospitals is that they cost so much. Hospitals often appear to be immune to many of the competitive forces of the normal marketplace, and thus regulation is proposed as a way to force them to contain their costs. In order to discuss the rapid increase in regulatory efforts, we must first understand why hospitals are less concerned than most industries with the cost of doing business.

For most products, interactions between manufacturers and consumers determine the price of the product and the amount that is sold. Consumers express their preferences in the marketplace by their decisions to buy. Firms compete with one another by advertising, by increasing quality or the appearance thereof, by cutting costs, by enlarging their factories and realizing economies of scale, and by investing in new capital equipment to improve efficiency. The consumer is the ultimate arbiter of this process, and the aggregate decisions of all consumers fix the value of the product and the price at which it can be sold.

Few markets in the modern world operate perfectly. External constraints imposed by government, monopolistic arrangements forged by business, and powerful labor unions distort the mechanism of the market. The hospital industry is an extreme example of a case where the market works poorly. That is, consumer preferences, at least in the short run, have little to do with what a hospital produces or how much its services cost. Patients have little choice as to what happens to the money that they spend purchasing hospital services.

To understand the genesis of this market failure, we must look at the way hospitals are organized, the signals to which they respond, and the goals to which they aspire. The first and foremost cause of market failure is hospital insurance, which insulates the consumer from the costs of purchasing hospital services. The vast majority of all hospital charges are paid by third parties on the behalf of consumers. Although these premiums are ultimately the responsibility of the consumer—either directly or through an employer or the government—patients rarely pay for more than a fraction of their hospital bills at the time services are received. This distance between the patient and the payment leaves consumers with the mistaken impression that they have very little economic stake in the efficiency of the hospital industry or the appropriateness of the hospital product.[15]

The dominance of the hospital industry by insurance does not in itself eliminate competition among hospitals. Third-party payers—insurance companies and government entities, for the most part—seek to promote efficiency in the industry in order to lower tax rates or insurance premiums. However, numerous other factors render price competition almost nonexistent. Hospitals, unlike other industries, are subject to stringent regulation and licensing requirements. There are substantial entry barriers to organizations that wish to compete in the hospital market. Certificate of need regulations prevent new hospitals from entering saturated markets even if these new entries would be able to produce comparable services at lower prices. Limitations on the numbers of available physicians and other skilled manpower also frustrate attempts to build alternative systems of care. Medicare and Medicaid further buffer hospitals from the consequences of inefficiency. The result is that existing hospitals rarely have to worry about the price they charge.

Another factor that frustrates market forces is the consumer's relative passivity. Most patients are neither able nor willing to make judgments about the kind of medical care they receive. Medical care is intrinsically complex and confusing, and the average person is unable to determine whether or not a given medical service is required. The physician is given the responsibility for making this choice. Moreover, at the moment most people require hospital care they are least capable of making slow and careful decisions about the services they are purchasing.

The situation is aggravated by the fee-for-service system, which gives both the hospital and the physician an incentive to produce more complex and costly medical services. Insurance companies usually pay bills on the basis of "usual, customary, and reasonable" charges. Such a standard allows hospitals to continually expand their services, secure in the knowledge that they can recover their investment through higher prices. The fact that the majority of hospitals are nonprofit does not diminish the desire of a hospital's governing board to expand its share of the market or the scope and cost of its product. This fact merely adds one more element that tends to make the hospital industry less sensitive to the costs it incurs and the prices it charges and helps to explain why hospital costs have escalated so rapidly.

Given that hospitals rarely compete on the basis of prices and are relatively indifferent to profit considerations, how do they set their institutional goals? For the most part, hospitals seek to maximize output: Bigger is better, and Cadillac care is preferred to the more pedestrian variety. This parallels the previous observations by Berry that hospitals go through a predictable and unidirectional evolutionary pattern. The trouble with this mode of operation is that it is impossible to know whether or not the consumer indeed prefers to spend four percent of the gross national product on hospitals. It is possible that consumers would rather spend a portion of the more than 50 billion dollars paid to hospitals to improve education, or perhaps just to purchase larger houses. Because the hospital industry is somewhat insulated from consumer decisions, it is highly likely that the current spectrum of available hospital services is excessive from the standpoint of consumer preference.

The unique role of the physician further heightens the distortions. Physicians purchase care on behalf of patients, without sharing any fiscal responsibility for the cost of the services they order.[28] Conversely, the more hospitalization, tests, and procedures physicians order, the higher their fees. In an era in which the penalty for error or a poor result may be a malpractice suit, physicians can diminish their risks at the insurer's cost by burying their uncertainty under a barrage of often superfluous tests. Thus, the incentives that play on hospital and physician are complementary and could be expected to combine to generate unnecessary utilization and high costs.

Many factors play a role in how hospitals are utilized in addition to treatment of patient illness. A variety of studies show that the supply of hospital beds and the number and type of available physicians exert a very strong influence on what hospitals do.[29-31] One graphic example is the observation by Wennberg and Gittlesohn that health care utilization in the state of Vermont varied tremendously from county to county, and that the observed differences had no relation to underlying patterns of illness or demography.[32] The authors note, "Hospitalization rates for specific admitting diagnoses and for surgical procedures are almost ten times greater in some hospital service areas as others. . . . The supply of surgeons is positively related to the surgery rate at all levels of surgical complexity and for nearly all types of individual procedures. Populations served by proportionately higher numbers of general practitioners performing surgery tend to have lower surgery rates for the more complex procedures and higher rates for the less complex procedures."

Other external factors also play a role in the way hospitals operate, and it is worth identifying several of the most important. One of these factors is the source of payment of the hospital bill. Studnicki found in Maryland that Medicaid patients stayed in the hospital significantly longer than patients covered by Blue Cross: 10.8 versus 8.3 days on the average for similar patients with similar diagnoses.[33] The differences could not be attributed to variations in the intensity of care provided or the severity of illness of the patients involved. He concludes that "whatever the mechanism, hospitals have apparently developed their own special variety of break-even dynamics in which the composition of the patient population by payment source exerts an extremely powerful influence."[33] Since the hospitals are almost totally dependent on third-party payers for reimbursement, it makes sense that they and the physicians might consciously or unconsciously discriminate among different coverages their patients carry and treat each patient somewhat differently to maximize the total revenue in each case.

Rural and urban differences may themselves affect the utilization of hospitals. In a study of the incidence of pediatric admissions among Medicaid recipients in the state of Washington, Connell observed marked variations in the hospital admission rates between rural and urban areas.[34] Urban counties tended to have higher surgical admissions, particularly for ear, nose, and throat (ENT) surgery, and rural counties tended to have more medical admissions. The author speculates that in rural areas hospitals may be used to substitute for ambulatory care, which may make sense considering the smaller number of physicians and more scattered population of rural areas. Horne, in a study of cholecystectomies in Saskatchewan, noted that length of stay was two days longer in areas where patients had to travel to obtain care, again reflecting the impact of residence on inpatient utilization patterns.[35] Other studies demonstrate that ambulatory care and inpatient care can theoretically substitute for each other in certain cases.[36,37] Although this is a complex issue, the volume and type of inpatient care consumed are affected by many factors beyond simple medical necessity.

The implications of this fact are profound for hospitals in general and rural hospitals in particular. Insurers and government bodies believe that they purchase excessive hospital services on behalf of their clients. Since there are few internally generated restraints on the growth in the hospital industry, government agencies and to some extent third-party payers have been striving to apply constraints from outside. These regulatory strictures surround the hospital industry and have increased rapidly. Their impact on the rural hospital is disproportionately severe, as we will discuss in the next section.

REGULATION, PLANNING, AND THE RURAL HOSPITAL

The major tools used by government bodies to mold the health service delivery system are planning and regulation. These take many forms. In the hospital industry government has concentrated on attempts to control the supply of hospital beds and has used reimbursement policies to shape hospital function. The vehicles through which these control mechanisms are applied are multiple. The major recent addition to the repertoire was Public Law 93–461, which erected a nationwide health planning structure with theoretically pervasive powers over hospital modifications. Medicare and Medicaid have always wielded great power by virtue of their control over a substantial portion of the total dollars flowing to hospitals. Although not a regulatory system, Medicare decisions have the effect of regulations. State governments, in general, have elaborate systems to accredit and license hospitals and have established a wide range of standards that cover issues ranging from the staffing requirements for obstetrical units down to the hardware needed in the hospital kitchen. The common denominator of all these attempts is that they exist because of the implicit recognition that hospitals as a class have little incentive to regulate their own cost or behavior.

Unfortunately, for the most part the regulatory effort has been disjointed, piecemeal, and ineffective, reflecting the disparate and at times mutually exclusive goals pursued by regulatory agencies. Because there is no logical foundation to the way in which hospital services are distributed nor any logical goals against which proposed modifications can be measured, the existing regulatory structure is cumbersome and often internally contradictory. In addition, despite the far-reaching powers granted to a variety of regulatory agencies by state and federal governments, regulators such as the Health Systems Agencies (HSAs) tend to act so as to maintain the status quo. This confluence of interest between the regulator and the regulated serves to further distort the normal market forces.

An excellent example of the regulatory process gone awry is the simplistic attempt to control utilization of hospital services by a formulaic approach to the supply of hospital beds. In a report published in 1976, the Institute of Medicine proclaimed that the source of the escalation of hospital costs lay in the increasing number of hospital beds per thousand population. The report noted that the supply of hospital beds had increased from 3.6 beds per thousand in 1960 to 4.4 beds per thousand in 1975. Acting on the observation that empty beds tend to be filled, the Committee recommended that the supply of hospital beds be decreased nationally to four per thousand.[38] This idea was echoed in a subsequent report commissioned by the federal government.[39]

Although the observation that hospital administrators and physicians act as if they abhor an empty hospital bed may have some basis in fact, regulations that set an arbitrary standard for total hospital bed supply are oversimplified and meddlesome. The observation that, in the aggregate, excessive hospital beds foster unnecessary utilization does not lead to the conclusion that the most effective way to reduce unnecessary utilization is to set an arbitrary figure for total supply. It is a very blunt and insensitive tool when applied to decisions about individual facilities. It ignores local conditions, historical patterns, and regional networks and frustrates more innovative approaches to the rationalization of hospital planning.

An example of this methodology misused in the hands of state health planners appears in an article by Walsh and Bicknell in which they promulgate a method for forecasting the need for hospital beds in Massachusetts. Instead of actually trying to determine how many hospital services are needed, they retrospectively use an arbitrary bed supply standard to justify reducing the supply of hospital beds. In a planning process whose entire goal is to restrain costs by restricting beds, it is deceptive to claim an internal logic for the method applied. The authors themselves note, "We reject as impractical the inductive method of building from morbidity data to a finding of needs for beds and used instead age-specific admissions as a proxy for hospital disability days. Theoretically these data can be predicted from detailed morbidity statistics, but realistically the data are not available in sufficient aggregation to be useful. . . ."[40]

The application of this approach is particularly pernicious for the individual rural hospital, where size and occupancy rate are related. Smaller hospitals maintain lower occupancy rates because of the statistical fluctuation in daily census. A standard that allocates beds to a rural county on the basis of its population will of necessity understate the number of beds needed if the towns are widely separated and the hospitals small.

Numerous other regulatory efforts are being applied or have been attempted. Currently, HSAs have statutory authority through certificate of need legislation to review and approve or disapprove all sizable modifications, improvements, or additions in hospitals within their purview. Although this has a certain inherent logic, in practice the review tends to perpetuate disparities in the delivery system. Large, affluent hospitals can afford to hire planners to prepare applications and argue the cases before the relevant HSAs. Larger hospitals have the depth of administrative staff and are located near the planning bodies. It is easier for them to develop personal relationships with the regulators and argue their cases more effectively.

In general, success of the regulatory process has been minimal, and its effect on rural hospitals has been deleterious.[41] Regulations tend to trigger survival behavior on the part of the institutions on whom they are imposed and may actually frustrate meaningful cooperation.[42] Regulatory agencies tend to increase the administrative costs of running hospitals. This is most noticeable in smaller hospitals in which there is limited administrative depth.[43] Despite a weighty regulatory apparatus, there is no evidence that it has helped to restrain costs. Feldstein notes, "Health planning has been a conservative approach to improving hospital performance. It has left unchanged the method used to reimburse hospitals and it has not changed the incentives facing physicians and hospitals and patients. . . . Health planning agencies have failed to improve the allocation of resources in the delivery of medical care. Even more costly, however, is the regulatory structure that has been created and will be difficult to remove."[10]

In many ways modifications in the reimbursement system show the greatest promise for controlling hospital behavior. Since a major cause of hospital inefficiency and irrational operations lies in the relative immunity of hospitals from the financial constraints of a normal market, efforts to create a market environment might yield major effects. We have discussed prospective reimbursement earlier in this chapter. Many states have embarked on this route. It is still too early in the process to forecast the results. Health Maintenance Organizations and various types of prepaid group practices have demonstrated their ability to lower health care costs by decreasing hospitalization rates. However, these organizations in general require large subscriber populations and have not proven to be very applicable to rural areas, with a few exceptions.[44] Medicare, Medicaid, and private insurance companies have all attempted to control costs but to date have been largely ineffective in changing hospital behavior. Medicare and Medicaid, beset by numerous regulations that set rigid and inflexible standards for the way hospitals must run and account for their costs, have actually heightened rural hospital difficulties by requiring compliance with standards that have little relevance to actual quality or efficiency.

One of the major political trends apparent in the 1980s is an attempt to dismantle much of the federally mandated regulatory apparatus coupled with an effort to stimulate competitive forces in the marketplace. The current administration is seeking to terminate the entire health planning process and use market forces as a way to determine the shape of the health care system. From the standpoint of the rural hospital, such changes will probably be welcome. Regulations have not proved to be very effective in meeting their objectives of constraining cost, and they have proved to be burdensome and, at times, contradictory. Whether or not it is possible to restore a normally functioning marketplace in the health sector is questionable, but rural hospitals should be able to adapt and compete successfully under such a concept.

OPTIONS AND STRATEGIES AVAILABLE TO THE RURAL HOSPITAL

The rural hospital often finds itself in a reactive posture, forced to respond to crises that are created by sudden changes in government policy, unanticipated loss of manpower, or financial difficulties. In this section we will review some of the options that may help rural hospitals to create more stable operating environments and better serve their communities. Only by anticipating change and developing mechanisms to cope with change can rural hospitals gain some control over the powerful external forces that impinge upon them. The ability of rural hospitals to grow and develop in a way consistent with the needs and aspirations of the local community will depend partially on the extent to which they use these strategies.

MULTI-INSTITUTIONAL ARRANGEMENTS

One way in which hospitals have tried to contain costs has been through the creation of various multi-institutional arrangements.

These arrangements run the gamut, from informal sharing of narrowly defined services to multihospital chains with centralized ownership and management.[45] Although the vast majority of these arrangements have been initiated by hospitals themselves, the promise of such approaches has been appreciated by federal regulators and incorporated in the guidelines promulgated for the National Health Planning and Resources Development Act of 1975.[46]

The logic behind multihospital arrangements lies in the perception that economies of scale exist in certain aspects of the hospital industry. The clearest example is shared purchasing arrangements. Small hospitals that purchase supplies in common can realize sizable volume discounts and have more clout with the various manufacturers. It has been estimated that 20 percent can be saved through shared purchasing agreements.[47]

The range of potential shared services is large, and a variety of ad hoc and formal affiliation arrangements have emerged. Among the variables that could be used for categorizing these affiliation arrangements are the degree of physical or organizational integration, legal bonds, the nature of services that are combined, the geography of populations served, and the organizational impact.[48] A useful way to categorize multihospital arrangements according to corporate ownership, corporate management, and system influence on major policy decisions is depicted in Figure 6.4. The seven major categories of multihospital arrangements include:[49]

1. *Formal affiliations.*   Two or more hospitals operate a single program, with each responsible for individual parts of the program.
2. *Shared or cooperative services.*   Clinical or administrative functions common to two or more organizations and used jointly or cooperatively for the purpose of improving service, effecting economies of scale, or both.
3. *Consortium.*   Formed when a group of hospitals agree to multiple affiliations. The hospitals work together to allocate programs and resources within the consortium.
4. *Contract management.*   Several hospitals are operated by an outside agency, group, or corporation but retain their boards and ownership.
5. *Lease.*   Policy, as well as field management, is provided by a separate corporate board or agency.

Types or Categories / Characteristics	I Formal Affiliation	II Shared or Cooperative Services	III Consortia for Planning or Education	IV Contract Management	V Lease	VI Corporate Ownership but Separate Management	VII Complete Ownership
	Less commitment, more institutional autonomy ———→ CONTINUUM ———→ More commitment, more system control						
Descriptions, definitions, terms	Patient transfer agreements; house officer affiliations; referral agreements	Financial, political commitment over time for selected products or services	Voluntary health planning council for a specific geography; Area Health Education Centers (AHECs)	Corporate management; full management without ownership	Policy as well as management provided by a single board	Owners do not interfere in the management of hospitals even though they have legal authority; absentee ownership	1. Mergers, consolidations 2. Satellites, branch operations 3. Authorities, chains 4. Holding companies
Corporate ownership	No	No	No	No	No	Yes	Yes
Corporate management	No	No	No	Yes	Yes	No	Yes
System influence on major policy decisions	No	No	Yes	Minor	Yes	Maybe	Yes (Absolute)

Figure 6.4. Classification of multihospital arrangements. (DeVries R: Strength in numbers. *Hospitals* 52:81–84, 1978. Reprinted with permission from *Hospitals, JAHA*, published by the American Hospital Association, copyright March 16, 1978, Vol. 52, No. 8.)

6. *Corporate ownership with separate management.* Reverse of a lease, in that a corporation owns a system of hospitals, but contracts for administration of each through separate boards.

7. *Complete ownership.* Common types include (a) mergers in which two or more institutions are joined together into a single body, with each institution relinquishing its corporate identity; (b) satellites resulting from a merger or the establishment of a branch operation by an existing institution; (c) hospital chains that are multiunit operations owned and operated by a central corporate body.

There are many instructive examples of how these multi-institutional arrangements work in the real world. The most widespread format involves shared services. Table 6.5 shows that the majority of hospitals in this country now participate in some sort of shared services agreement, and the number is rising. It is interesting to note that smaller hospitals are those least likely to participate, although theoretically they would most benefit from pooling their strength. Those services that are shared remain rather limited, and of the 10 most common shared services, only three are clinical: blood bank, laboratory/pathology, and radiology.[50] Various purchasing arrangements of drugs, food, laundry services, and a variety of supplies remain by far the most common shared activity. With the exception of the three clinical categories mentioned, no clinical area shows much evidence of shared operations. It is clear that hospitals remain wary of submerging their identity in larger hospital networks. Consortia to run continuing medical education and agreements to purchase linen in common are acceptable, but arrangements that yield control and autonomy to some central power are not.

An example of an acceptable arrangement is the Virginia Mason Consortium involving Virginia Mason Hospital, a large tertiary care facility in Seattle, Washington, and 10 small rural hospitals in the state of Washington.[51] The average size of Virginia Mason Consortium hospitals is 49 beds, and they are located 76 to 160 miles from Seattle.[48] Each member hospital defines its own needs and programs and pays for the services it requests. Educational programs involve physicians, trustees, administration, and the nursing, dietary, medical records, and engineering staffs. In addition to education

TABLE 6.5. Participation in Shared Services by Short-Term Community General Hospitals by Bed Size, 1975 and 1978

Bed Size	1975			1978		
	Number Surveyed	Number Participating	Percentage Participating	Number Surveyed	Number Participating	Percentage Participating
6–99	2,430	1,312	54.0	2,123	1,662	78.3
100–199	1,208	795	65.8	1,157	1,012	87.5
200–299	592	438	74.0	618	555	89.8
300–399	364	287	78.8	345	320	92.8
400–499	212	170	80.2	219	202	92.2
500 or more	268	207	77.2	282	255	90.4
Total	5,074	3,209	63.2	4,744	4,006	84.4

Source: Taylor, Elworth: Survey shows who is sharing which services. *Hospitals* 53:147–152, 1979, Table 2. Reprinted with permission, from *Hospitals, Journal of the American Hospital Association*, published by the American Hospital Association, copyright September 16, 1979, Vol. 53, No. 18.

programs, the consortium has developed a cooperative medical audit program and a series of health education forums and has provided assistance in the recruitment of physicians, nurses, and laboratory and x-ray personnel. From Virginia Mason's perspective, the primary benefit of the consortium is the increase in patient referrals to the tertiary care hospital.

A number of other useful multi-institutional arrangements exist. Carolina Hospital and Health Services, Inc. (CHHS) was initiated by the state hospital associations of North and South Carolina in 1969 and is a freestanding, nonprofit, shared services corporation. CHHS provides a variety of services to hospitals, including management engineering, biomedical instrumentation, affiliated purchasing program, claims collection bureau, facilities development, and comprehensive management contract services.[48] The contract management services are provided by CHHS for a fixed sum of money, but the hospital, through its board of governors, retains total control of the institution. CHHS emphasizes the development of appropriate financial management systems for the small rural hospital.

Rural hospitals often lack sufficient management expertise to cope with the diversity of administrative problems that they must face due to increasingly complex planning, regulatory, and reimbursement processes as well as the dynamics of internal staff relationships. There are no career ladders for management in small rural hospitals, and it is often difficult to be able to attract or afford capable administrative staff. Contract management programs are, therefore, attractive to rural hospitals with management problems and a desire to retain their institutional autonomy.[52]

Health Central, Inc. is a not-for-profit, health care management and service organization with headquarters in Minneapolis. Health Central, Inc., has provided a range of sharing programs and services for rural hospitals throughout the upper Midwest and has affiliations with over 100 hospitals and nursing homes as well as owning or operating 11 health care institutions. Health Central is a good example of a large multihospital system that tries to tailor its services to the individual needs of a rural hospital. In addition to negotiating over 250 contracts involving more than 10,000 supply items, Health Central has affiliation agreements with three hospitals under which they provide a complete set of shared services, management contracts with two hospitals, and two small rural hospitals that are corporate members.[47]

An interesting example of multihospital systems that exert greater system control are the investor-owned hospital chains that have rapidly developed during the past decade. In 1973, for-profit hospitals operated 24 hospitals under management contracts; this number grew to 250 hospitals by 1978.[53] Investor-owned chains have tended to compete on their own terms—they have generally operated in rural areas and single hospital communities where little or no competition existed. Investor-owned chains have the capability of being able to preserve, accumulate, and attract capital and recently have made strong efforts to acquire small rural hospitals located in rapid growth areas.[54]

A recent report indicates that investor-owned chains are starting to compete with not-for-profit multihospital systems for market share in the state of Utah.[55] Hospital Corporation of America, the largest for-profit multihospital system, and Intermountain Health Care, a successful not-for-profit hospital chain, are competing with each other, but not on the basis of price. Instead, their competition focuses on facility attractiveness to physicians and ability to offer the most sophisticated technology.

As these examples demonstrate, there are many ways in which rural hospitals can become involved in multi-institutional arrangements. The advantage of joining together with other hospitals is that there is strength in numbers, and costs can often be lowered by sharing services or by common purchasing. The disadvantages are loss of flexibility and autonomy. Rural hospitals have the opportunity to investigate a spectrum of possible affiliation mechanisms. As an increasing number of larger corporate organizations become interested in acquiring or affiliating with smaller hospitals, rural communities can be more selective in their choice of partners.

DIVERSIFICATION OF SERVICES

Hospital diversification has been defined as the conscious attempt to expand the range of services of a hospital both to meet community needs and to improve utilization of the hospital resources, thereby providing a stable financial base.[56] Golda lists the following prerequisites for successful diversification:

1. Effective long-range planning
2. Community participation
3. Market analysis
4. Favorable political and regulatory climate
5. Flexible management philosophy
6. Recognition of the risk of failure

The range of diversification options available to the rural hospital depends on the spectrum of services that can be provided, the setting for the services, and the segment of the population to be served. The rural hospital can either be directly or indirectly involved with service diversification.[57] Examples of direct involvement include independently providing services, acting as a vendor under terms of a contract, and developing a partnership with other health facilities; indirect involvement would have the hospital acting as an organizer, facilitator, or a change agent that induced other providers to get involved in diversification strategies. Rural hospitals have the opportunity to become human services centers that are the focal point for broadly diversified human services.[56]

One of the critical elements of a successful diversification program is an appropriate marketing strategy. Flexner and Berkowitz[58] urge that marketing research methods be incorporated into the institutional planning process. MacStravic has found that all new program opportunities require extensive marketing analysis in contrast to the more traditional inpatient programs that rely mainly on physician recruitment.[59] Institutional resource allocation decisions should be guided by consumer needs and wants, rather than the opposite. Therefore, any diversification strategy should be associated with a particular market segment of consumers.

The marketing concept should be viewed as a systematic approach, rather than a "quick fix." Its goal is to introduce consumer needs as the focal point for institutional planning and decision making. This type of approach can lead to successful institutional decisions concerning the introduction of new services that are responsive to the needs of consumers, providers, and the community in general.

Three of the diversification strategies that have been used by rural hospitals are: the delivery of primary care, the establishment of health maintenance organizations (HMOs), and the use of swing-

beds to provide long-term care services. We have discussed the first
two options extensively in Chapter 4 and will not repeat the discussion here. Both options offer opportunities for rural hospitals to
expand their service base and modify their organizational
frameworks, but both also involve significant developmental costs
and risks. They should be considered carefully by rural hospitals
seeking to increase their market share or broaden their scope of
services.

The adoption of the swing-bed concept may have more general
applicability for rural hospitals than either the primary care or HMO
options. Rural areas are often faced with inadequate health care facilities for their sizable elderly populations. Nonmetropolitan counties have a high proportion (13 percent) of elderly residents but have
only half of the number of skilled nursing home beds per 1,000
elderly as do metropolitan counties.[60] One response to this problem
has been the use of swing-beds to provide long-term care services to
the rural elderly.

Swing-beds are hospital beds that can be used to provide care to
either acute or long-term care patients.[61] The swing-bed concept has
developed in response to the high occupancy rates of certified rural
nursing homes and the declining volume of patient days experienced
by many rural hospitals. It is an approach that will hopefully improve
the financial viability and community image of the rural hospital and
also improve the ability of rural communities to provide long-term
care in their local environment.

Proponents of the swing-bed approach assume that:[62]

1. Unmet demand for institutional long-term care exists in rural
   communities.
2. Rural hospitals with low occupancy rates have surplus staff capacity.
3. With sufficient training, hospital staff members can provide adequate long-term care.
4. Rural hospitals can provide institutional long-term care in a cost-
   effective manner.
5. The swing-bed approach can markedly decrease travel costs for
   long-term care patients and family members.
6. Rural communities have a strong need to maintain their local
   hospital.

In the past, rural hospitals rarely used swing-beds to provide long-term care for the elderly. Medicare and Medicaid required that hospitals be certified to provide long-term care if they were to be reimbursed for these services. Certification meant that hospitals providing long-term care offer a variety of services, including physical therapy, social services, and patient activities. These services are not routinely provided by many rural hospitals, and this discouraged some facilities from utilizing the swing-bed concept. Regulations also required the provision of long-term care in a physically distinct part of a hospital, exclusively set aside for such purposes. This regulation was developed to insure that a hospital would appropriately report its costs associated with the provision of long-term care. It effectively reduced the ability of rural hospitals to use their supply of beds efficiently in meeting the needs of their acute and long-term care patients.

In the mid-1970s, the federal government funded swing-bed experiments in the states of Utah, Texas, South Dakota, and Iowa. One hundred eight rural hospitals participated in this study, and a well-designed evaluation of the pros and cons of providing long-term care in rural hospitals was initiated. Key features of the experiment were (1) waiver of Medicare and Medicaid conditions of participation and (2) reimbursement on a per-diem basis rather than on the standard cost basis commonly used by Medicare, with an incentive payment to encourage participation in the program.

The overall policy recommendation of the study was the implementation of a national swing-bed program in rural communities.[62] This recommendation was based on (1) the existence of unmet demand for long-term care in rural areas, (2) the belief that appropriate quality assurance programs would enable rural hospitals to provide adequate long-term care, and (3) the finding that the cost of swing-bed care is less than the cost of similar care provided in other institutional settings, although no comparisons were made with non-institutional alternatives.[63]

The results of this study helped lay the groundwork for the passage of federal legislation on swing-beds. Section 904 of the Omnibus Reconciliation Act of 1980 allows rural hospitals with fewer than 50 beds to provide long-term care services to Medicare beneficiaries and Medicaid recipients if the hospitals have certificates of need for the provision of these services and they offer discharge planning and social services. Rural hospitals will be reimbursed at the average rate per patient day paid under a state's Title 19 plan for routine services to nursing homes.[64]

It makes sense for rural hospitals to broaden the base of services that they offer to their communities. Diversification allows more extensive use of the existing capital plant and hospital personnel, builds community support, and meets important human needs. Although not without risk, diversification of services can strengthen the economic status of the rural hospital by spreading the cost of hospital operation over a wider spectrum of activities and attracting new revenue. Each rural hospital should evaluate existing unmet health and social needs within its medical service area and consider the possibility of using the hospital as an institutional focus for meeting those needs.

REGIONALIZATION OF HOSPITAL SERVICES

Regionalization is a valuable planning concept that has been blurred and misused over the last 20 years. Regionalization is based on a systems approach toward the provision of medical services. It grows from the recognition that it is impossible and undesirable to provide all conceivable services that a given population requires in one place. Regionalization implies that services within a specific geographic region will be coordinated and that each health institution within that region will provide those services that are appropriate to the population it serves, its location, and its capabilities. With regard to inpatient services, rural hospitals will provide basic ambulatory and inpatient services, and urban hospitals will act as referral centers for complex, expensive, and risky procedures.

Regionalization has been confused with centralization, in which *all* medical services are provided in central, usually urban locations. In a logical regional delivery system, certain procedures are centralized because they are performed infrequently or require expensive technology or highly specialized personnel. By the same token, however, primary care services are decentralized so that they are available to people where they live and provided by health professionals whom they know. The blurring of the distinction between regionalization and centralization has had the perverse effect of undermining the capability of rural hospitals to provide basic ser-

TABLE 6.6. Surgical Operations and Size of Hospital, United States, 1976

Bed Size of Hospital	All Discharges	Without Surgery	With Surgery	Percent of Discharges with Surgery
6–99	6,594	4,714	1,880	28.5
100–199	5,701	3,531	2,170	38.1
200–299	5,389	3,053	2,336	43.4
300–499	9,355	5,074	4,281	45.8
500+	7,332	3,756	3,577	48.8
Totals	34,371	20,127	14,244	41.4

Source: *Utilization of Short-Stay Hospitals: Annual Summary for the United States, 1976.* Vital and Health Statistics Series 13–Number 37. USDHEW, DHEW Pub. No. (PHS) 78–1788, June 1978, Table E.

vices. Regulation has tended to spur centralization, often as an unanticipated side effect of the cumulative weight of multiple regulations.

Our current health care system is already highly centralized. Tables 6.6 through 6.8 depict the relation between hospital size and the type and amount of inpatient care in the United States. In Table 6.6 we observe that surgical procedures are a much larger component of the activities of larger hospitals and account for only 28.5 percent of the discharges in the hospital size range where most rural hospitals fall. In Table 6.7 we see that the most common discharge diagnoses for small hospitals are different than those for hospitals as a whole. Although we cannot directly infer that smaller hospitals care for less complex inpatient problems, the distribution of discharge diagnoses would favor that conclusion. Table 6.8 depicts the types of surgical procedures that are performed by small and large hospitals, and the disparity is even more apparent than for the diagnostic groupings. It is apparent that small hospitals have restricted their scope of surgical operations to those with the least complexity. Although the surgical listings are relatively broad, all the operations that are frequently performed in small hospitals are common procedures with low mortality rates. This is in marked contrast to larger hospitals, whose surgical repertoire is skewed much more toward complex and dangeous procedures. This is an entirely appropriate pattern if we bear in mind the data presented by Luft et al.[25]

Most regionalization has occurred without explicit regulatory in-

TABLE 6.7. Most Common Discharge Diagnoses for Smallest and Largest U.S. Hospitals, 1976

Diagnosis	Small Hospitals (6–99 Beds)		Large Hospitals (>500 Beds)		All Hospitals	
	Rank Order	*% of All Diagnoses*	*Rank Order*	*% of All Diagnoses*	*Rank Order*	*% of All Diagnoses*
Diseases of respiratory system	1	14	6	7	5	10
Disease of digestive system	2	14	4	10	2	12
Diseases of circulatory system	3	14	2	12	1	13
Accidents, poisoning, and violence	4	11	5	10	4	10
Complications of pregnancy, childbirth, puerperium	5	9	1	12	3	12
Totals		62		51		57

Source: *Utilization of Short-Stay Hospitals: Annual Summary for the United States, 1976. Vital and Health Statistical Series 13–Number 37.* USDHEW, DHEW Pub. No. (PHS) 78-1788, June 1978, Table 21.

tervention. Attempts to force regionalization can become a convenient excuse to shut down small or rural hospitals and cluster all hospital services in central urban locations. A blatant example of the misuse of the concept of regionalization occurred in relation to the regulations issued to implement the National Health Planning Act referred to earlier. The most potentially disruptive part of those regulations dealt with obstetric care. The first draft of the regulations stated, "Facilities not located in SMSAs of over 100,000 population should provide at least 500 deliveries annually. . . . Below 500 deliveries, the quality of care and efficiency are decreased significantly."[65] This regulation brought an enormous outcry from throughout rural America; its implementation would have closed the majority of obstetric units in rural America. The impact on rural communities would have been far reaching and disruptive. Particularly in an era when family-centered noninterventionist obstetrics is becoming the standard, this regulation would have forced almost all rural women who desired a hospital delivery to travel to regional centers to deliver their children, far from friends and family.

The irony of the proposed regulation is that it is not based on fact. In a study of obstetric quality in rural Iowa, Hein found that the neonatal death rate in rural hospitals was lower than that found in urbanized portions of the state.[66] Obstetric care in Iowa had been regionalized from within and appropriate transfer of high risk mothers and infants is a reality. Similar work in California has shown only marginally higher infant mortality rates in rural hospitals, after correction for sociodemographic status of the populations at risk.[67] Closing of all rural obstetric units would have destroyed rather than fostered regionalization and raised rather than lowered costs.

Sensitive and sensible regionalization is a useful and realistic objective for the rural community. A useful tool in helping to determine which services can be provided locally and which should be regionalized is the travel time standard. Rural hospitals can best define their medical service area—and thus their target populations—in terms of those people who live within a reasonable travel distance of the hospital. This makes sense because the use of health services is determined to a certain extent by the distance one must travel to obtain them. Hospital services are no exception, and people dislike having to travel long distances to obtain inpatient care. In addition to the expense incurred, one must take into account the

TABLE 6.8. Relative Frequency of Selected Surgical Operations Performed in Large and Small Short-Stay Hospitals, United States, 1976

Surgical Category and ICDA Code	Small Hospitals (6–99 Beds)		Large Hospitals (>500 Beds)		All Hospitals	
	Rank Order	% of Total Operations	Rank Order	% of Total Operations	Rank Order	% of Total Operations
Plastic surgery (92–94)	1	8.3	3	4.9	2	5.4
Dilation and curettage of uterus (70.3)	2	4.9	4	4.2	3	4.9
Tonsillectomy (21.1–21.2)	3	4.8	13	1.7	6	3.1
Biopsy (A1–A2)	4	4.1	2	6.5	1	5.6
Inguinal herniorrhaphy (38.2–38.3)	5	3.1	7	2.0	7	2.5

Hysterectomy (69.1–69.5)	6	3.0	5	2.5	5	3.4
Appendectomy (41.1)	7	2.8	24	1.0	18	1.5
Tubal ligation (68.5)	8	2.8	9	1.9	10	2.1
Cholecystectomy (43.5)	9	2.7	10	1.8	9	2.2
Operations on muscle, tendons, etc. (88–89)	10	2.3	12	1.7	13	1.8
Vascular and cardiac (24–30)	19	1.3	1	8.0	4	4.8
Oophorectomy (67.2–67.5)	11	2.3	6	2.1	8	2.3
Caesarian section (77)	16	1.4	8	2.0	12	1.9

Source: *Utilization of Short-Stay Hospitals: Annual Summary for the United States, 1976.* Vital and Health Statistics, Series 13–Number 37. USDHEW, DHEW Pub. No. (PHS) 78-1788, June 1978, Table 27.

psychological costs of being hospitalized apart from community and friends. As England has pointed out, ". . . if rural populations are to receive some of the care they could benefit from, it must be provided much closer to where they live and in circumstances which they are culturally able to accept and financially able to support. This means that the primary health services must be able to provide as full a range as possible of locally needed services."[68]

Hospitals are located in population centers and draw their clientele from the surrounding area. The service areas of hospitals overlap at the periphery, and just like grocery stores or movie houses, hospitals compete for "customers." In general, there is an inverse relationship between the utilization of hospital services and the travel distance, with the shape of the relationship varying with the ease of travel. If you live far from a hospital and the roads are poor or transportation nonexistent, you may be reluctant or unable to seek needed help.[69]

The concept of distance as a key component of access has been officially recognized in the National Health Planning Guidelines that emerged as part of the process of operationalizing Public Law 93–641, the National Health Planning Act. In the section setting the allowable standards for hospital bed supply, rural areas are dealt with separately. "Hospital care should be accessible within a reasonable period of time. For example, in rural areas in which a majority of the residents would otherwise be more than 30 minutes travel time from a hospital, the HSA may determine, based on analyses, that a bed-population ratio of greater than four per thousand persons may be justified. Travel distance to the nearest hospital is one of the most important factors to be analyzed, especially in rural areas. A planning criteria of 30 minutes has been set, in line with the policies of many local and state health planning agencies around the country."[70]

This national recognition of a transportation isochrone, first proposed by Bridgman many years earlier,[71] gives us an operational tool with which to approach the planning of hospital services in rural areas, an approach we will explore further in Chapter 8. A transportation isochrone is a circumferential line around a population center whose position is determined by the amount of time taken to travel from the periphery to the center. The half-hour travel standard is arbitrary, but it establishes a method by which to define the catchment area for any given rural area. The travel standard also has the advantage of adapting to changes in the technology of transportation. The expansion of the national highway network has enlarged the circles around many rural towns and made it possible for larger segments of the dispersed rural population to obtain medical services. On the other hand, the rapidly increasing costs of energy may lead to a constriction of the circle when and if increasing segments of the rural population can no longer afford to operate private automobiles.

This transportation yardstick allows rural hospitals to determine their potential marketplace with some precision. A knowledge of the population age structure allows one to calculate the number of expected annual hospital admissions for specific conditions that will be required by the service area population. Sensible regionalization then becomes the process by which those admissions are partitioned between the rural hospital and other external facilities on the basis of relative cost and quality. In this way regionalization becomes a planning tool that the community can use to shape the future of its own medical services, not a set of dictates imposed from outside.

Regionalization can be a useful strategy for the rural hospital that is attempting to define its proper place in the health care delivery system. Regionalization has been occurring as a natural consequence of changes in the way medical care is produced and delivered. It is not uniform, or always logical, and undoubtedly there are examples of rural areas referring too little. However, it is just as likely that there are large segments of medical services not provided in rural areas because of inadequate hospitals or insufficient manpower that could be provided as safely and more cheaply at home than in a regional center. The challenge is to develop an approach to regionalization based on patient needs, rather than use regionalization as a technique to consolidate or eliminate all but large urban institutions.

THE PROSPECT FOR THE RURAL HOSPITAL

The rural hospital is not merely a smaller version of the urban hospital. Evidence supports the conclusion that rural hospitals play a different role in their communities than do urban hospitals of similar size. Rural hospitals are forced by their relative isolation to care for a wider variety of patients than small urban hospitals and are required to maintain the capability to care for emergency problems that do not permit ready transfer. For these reasons, rural hospitals may have to purchase certain items of equipment or maintain staffing that is relatively inefficient because it is infrequently used but necessary for the protection of the community.

Hospitals are under siege because they are seen as the engine in a rapid spiral of cost inflation in the medical field. Because the hospital industry is relatively insensitive to normal market constraints, government agencies have attempted to restrain escalating costs through external controls. Unfortunately, this regulatory exoskeleton has been constructed piecemeal and has been largely ineffective in accomplishing its aims. In fact, it can be persuasively argued that the bulk of the regulatory structure is inherently cost provocative and the cure is worse than the disease.

The prospect for rural hospitals is mixed. It is clear from the review of the evidence that rural hospitals are not necessarily more expensive than larger urban facilities. Size plays a relatively minor role in determining the ultimate cost of hospital care. When travel costs are considered, it appears highly likely that rural hospitals are intrinsically less expensive than urban hospitals. Since one of the major costs of hospital care lies in what services a hospital equips itself to do, it makes sense to build the industry around a cooperative network of small, decentralized facilities providing relatively basic levels of care. Closing rural hospitals forces costs to rise rapidly by shunting unselected, uncomplicated patients into secondary and tertiary centers where the technological capability exceeds the patients' medical needs.

The issue of quality is a crucial one in determining the fate of rural hospitals. Quality is directly related to the volume of a given procedure occurring in any given hospital. Each procedure or treatment protocol appears to have its own volume threshold, and it seems quite plausible to determine the minimum required volume needed to adequately care for a given condition. It is apparent that many of the "bread-and-butter" diagnoses can be cared for safely by rural hospitals.

Rural hospitals are threatened by government's inability or unwillingness to realize that rural hospitals form a special class. Regulations designed to curb costs, even if they are nonsensical or irrelevant, fall with a heavier weight on small hospitals. Although rural hospitals comprise a fairly large proportion of the total number of hospitals in the United States, they care for only a small fraction of the patients and generate an even smaller proportion of total costs. It would make sense to identify the rural hospital as a vital community resource and erect a regulatory structure that recognizes and supports this important role. If this is not done, the danger exists that rural hospitals will disappear and in so doing destroy the foundation upon which the rest of the rural health care system is based.

Rural hospitals must assume responsibility for charting their own future. The scope of services a rural hospital elects to provide has direct implications on both the quality of care and the economic viability of the institution. Rural hospitals must involve themselves in an internally generated planning process by which the services they offer become a reflection of the needs of the community and incorporate what we know about the relationship between the volume and quality of care. This approach towards planning, in which the spectrum of possible hospital services is partitioned between the rural community and other sources of care, is explored in detail in the last chapter.

The stresses upon the rural hospital will change during the next decade. Regulatory intensity will diminish somewhat as a result of a more laissez-faire political philosophy, but regulation will continue to be an important fact of life for rural hospitals. Attempts to constrain rising costs through the marketplace will have an unpredictable effect on the rural hospital. It is quite possible that rural hospitals that are able to provide care of adequate quality at reduced cost will recapture some of the market share that they lost over the last 30 years. Technological innovation will generate expensive new equipment that may or may not benefit patient care and justify its cost. On the other hand, some technological innovations, such as the minicomputer and rapid advances in communication, may significantly decrease the expense of improved diagnostic and management tools. One can only conclude that rural hospitals will continue to play a central role in rural health care systems but that they will have to retain flexibility to adapt to a rapidly changing and unpredictable future.

REFERENCES

1. Geyman JP: On the plight of the rural hospital. *Journal of Family Practice* 6:477–478, 1978.
2. Woolf M: Demographic factors associated with physician staffing in rural areas: The experience of the National Health Service Corps. *Medical Care* 19:444–451, 1981.
3. Cotterill PG, Eisenberg BS: Improving access to medical care in underserved areas: The role of group practice. *Inquiry* 16:141–153, 1979.
4. Sorenson AA, Kunitz SJ: The changing distribution of physicians in regionville. *Rural Sociology* 43:711–725, 1978.
5. Somers AR: *Health Care in Transition: Directions for the Future.* Chicago, Hospital Research and Educational Trust, 1970.
6. D'Elia G, Folse R, Robertson R: Family practice in nonmetropolitan Illinois. *Journal of Family Practice* 8:799–805, 1979.
7. Evans EO: New use for the smaller peripheral general hospital. *Lancet* 2:423–424, 1969.
8. McCarthy JB: A planning process for rural health care. *Hospital Forum* 19:7–8, 1976.
9. Berry RE: Cost and efficiency in the production of hospital services. *MMFQ* 52:291–313, 1974.
10. Feldstein PJ: *Health Care Economics.* New York. John Wiley and Sons, 1979.
11. Carr WJ, Feldstein PJ: The relationship of cost to hospital size. *Inquiry* 4:45–65, 1967.
12. Edwards M, Miller JD, Schumacher R: Classification of community hospitals by scope of service: Four indexes. *Health Services Research* 7:301–313, Winter 1972.
13. Zaretsky HW: The effects of patient mix and service mix on hospital costs and productivity. *Topics in Health Care Financing* 4:63–82, 1979.
14. Berry RE: Product heterogeneity and hospital cost analysis. *Inquiry* 7:67–75, 1970.
15. Klastorin T, Watts C, Trivedi V: *A Study of the Classification of Hospitals for Prospective Reimbursement.* Health Care Financing Research and Demonstrations Series, report no. 10, DHEW (HCFA), U.S. Government Printing Office, 620–010/4019, 1979.
16. Klastorin TD, Watts CA: On the measurement of hospital case mix. *Medical Care* 18:675–685, 1980.
17. Krischer JP: Indexes of severity: Underlying concepts. *Health Services Research* 11:143–157, 1976.

18. Lave JR, Lave LB: The extent of role differentiation among hospitals. *Health Services Research* 6:15–38, 1971.
19. Schumacher DN, Horn SD, Solnick MF, et al: Hospital cost per case. *Medical Care* 17:1037–1046, 1979.
20. Spitzer WO: The small general hospital. *MMFQ* 48:431–447, 1970.
21. Roemer MI: Is surgery safer in larger hospitals? *Hospital Management* 87:35–37, 1959.
22. Riedel DC, Fitzpatrick TB: *Patterns of Patient Care.* Ann Arbor, University of Michigan Press, 1964.
23. Moses LE, Mosteller F: Institutional differences in postoperative death rates: Commentary on some of the findings of the National Halothane Study. *Journal of the American Medical Association* 203:150–152, 1968.
24. Ashley JSA, Howlett A, Morris JN: Case-fatality of hyperplasia of the prostate in two teaching and three regional hospitals. *Lancet* 2:1308–1311, 1971.
25. Luft HS, Bunker JP, Enthoven AC: Should operations be regionalized? The empirical relation between surgical volume and mortality. *New England Journal of Medicine* 301:1363–1369, 1979.
26. Stroll JK, Willis PW, Reynolds EW, et al: Effectiveness of coronary care units in small community hospitals. *Annals of Internal Medicine* 95:709–713, 1976.
27. Flood AB, Ewy W, Scott WR, et al: The relationship between intensity and duration of medical services and outcomes for hospitalized patients. *Medical Care* 17:1088–1102, 1979.
28. Eisenberg JM, Rosoff AJ: Physician responsibility for the cost of unnecessary medical services. *New England Journal of Medicine* 299:76–80, 1978.
29. LoGerfo JP: Variation in surgical rates: Fact vs. fantasy. *New England Journal of Medicine* 297:387–388, 1977.
30. Lewis CE: Variations in the incidence of surgery *New England Journal of Medicine* 281:880–884, 1969.
31. Harris DM: Effect of population and health care environment on hospital utilization. *Health Services Research* 10:229–243, 1975.
32. Wennberg J, Gittelsohn A: Small area variations in health care delivery. *Science* 182:1102–1108, 1973.
33. Studnicki J: Differences in length of stay for Medicaid and Blue Cross patients and the effect of intensity of service. *Public Health Reports* 94:438–445, 1979.
34. Connell FA, Day RW, LoGerfo JP: Hospitalization of Medicaid children: Analysis of small area variations in admission rates. *American Journal of Public Health* 71:606–613, 1981.
35. Horne JM, Beck RG: Temporal patterns in the use of health services

leading to cholecystectomy: A process evaluation using insurance records. *Medical Care* 16:1006–1018, 1978.

36. Bellin SS, Geiger HJ, Gibson CD: Impact of ambulatory health care services on the demand for hospital beds. *New England Journal of Medicine* 280:808–812, 1969.

37. Mushlin AI, Appel FA: Extramedical factors in the decision to hospitalize medical patients. *American Journal of Public Health* 66:170–172, 1976.

38. *Controlling the Supply of Hospital Beds.* Institute of Medicine, National Academy of Sciences, Washington, D.C., October 1976.

39. McClure W: *Reducing excess hospital capacity.* National Technical Information Service, HRP–0015199, October 1976.

40. Walsh DC, Bicknell WJ: Forecasting the need for hospital beds: A quantitative methodology. *Public Health Reports* 92:199–210, 1977.

41. Peeples D: *Rural Community Health Facility Report.* Unpublished manuscript, Washington Alaska RMP, 1975.

42. Kinzer DM: Why health care regulation isn't working. *Trustee* 30:29–32, November 1977.

43. Kunitz SJ, Sorensen AA: The effects of regional planning on a rural hospital: A case study. *Social Science and Medicine* 13D:1–11, 1979.

44. Wheeler JR, Ackor JD: Should smaller hospitals operate HMOs? *Hospitals* 48:93–95, 1974.

45. Connors EJ: Multihospital systems are changing the health care landscape. *Trustee* 32:24–5, 28–30, 1979.

46. Mason SA: The multihospital movement defined. *Public Health Reports* 94:446–453, 1979.

47. Wegmiller DC: Multi-institutional pacts offer rural hospitals do-or-die options. *Hospitals* 52:52–54, 1978.

48. Zuckerman H: Multi-institutional systems: Promises and performance. *Inquiry*, 291–316, 1979.

49. Rice J: How to choose the right multihospital system. *Trustee* 34(1):17–21, 1981.

50. Taylor E: Survey shows who is sharing which services. *Hospitals* 53:147–150, 152, 1979.

51. Friedrich P, Ross A: Consortium serves rural hospitals' educational needs. *Hospitals* 51:95–96, 1977.

52. Childers B: *Contract Management in the Small Not for Profit Hospital.* Mimeo, Methodist Hospital of Indiana, 1977.

53. Mason S: The multihospital movement defined. *Public Health Reports* 94:446–453, 1979.

54. Di Paolo V: Investor-owned systems: For profits target smaller hospitals. *Modern Health Care* 10:86–87, 1980.

55. Brazda J (ed): Competition in Utah; The struggle has just begun. *Health*, p 8, June 1981.
56. Golda E: Rural hospital diversification strategies. *Health Care Planning and Marketing* 1:1–10, July 1981.
57. Melum M: Hospitals must change, control is the issue. *Hospitals* 54:67–72, 1980.
58. Flexner W, Berkowitz E: Marketing research in health services planning: A model. *Public Health Reports* 94:503–514, 1979.
59. MacStravic S: *Marketing by Objectives for Hospitals*. Germantown, Aspen Publications, 1980.
60. *Rural Hospital Program of Extended Care Services*. Princeton, NJ, Robert Wood Johnson Foundation, 1981.
61. *A Position Paper on Swing Bed Care in Hospitals*. Denver, Health Services Research Center, University of Colorado, 1978.
62. *An Evaluation of Swing Bed Experiments to Provide Long Term Care in Rural Hospitals*. Denver, Health Services Research Center, University of Colorado, 1980.
63. Newton A: Rural health care thrives under hospital's pre-paid plan. *Hospitals* 51:45–58, 1977.
64. *Swing bed provision of omnibus reconciliation act of 1980*. Small or Rural Hospitals Report, 1–2, AHA, Chicago, January–February 1981.
65. Hein H, Ferguson N: The cost of maternity care in rural hospitals. *Journal of the American Medical Association* 240:2051–2052, 1978.
66. Hein H: The quality of perinatal care in small rural hospitals. *Journal of the American Medical Association* 240:2070–2072, 1978.
67. Williams R: Measuring the effectiveness of perinatal medical care. *Medical Care* 17:110, 1979.
68. England R: A planned role for the hospital in rural areas. *World Hospital* 13:131–133, 1977.
69. Shannon GW, Bashshur RL, Metznerm CA: The concept of distance as a factor in accessibility and utilization of health care. *Medical Care Review* 26:143–161, 1969.
70. Johnson RL: Rural hospitals face change for a bright future. *Hospitals* 52:47–50, 1978.
71. Bridgman RF: *The Rural Hospital*. Geneva, WHO, 1955.

CHAPTER 7

Other Important
Rural Health Services:
Care for the Elderly,
Mental Health Care,
and Dental Care

The focus of this book thus far has been on health services directed primarily at acute medical problems: the provision of emergency, ambulatory, and hospital care. There are a variety of other health problems and matching health services that are important to the rural population. In this chapter we select three of these areas for further consideration: care for the elderly, mental health services, and dental care.

Over the last 20 years these three topics have received increasing attention from private and public sources, attention that has been accompanied by the creation of a significant number of governmentally sponsored programs designed to improve access to and the quality of services in these areas. These interventions have for the most part been national in scope, without a particular rural emphasis. The problems addressed by these programs are not limited to rural areas, although in each case there are certain aspects of the rural situation that require a tailor-made approach. As a result, specific data on the manifestation of the problem in rural areas are lacking,

228

and we are often forced to extrapolate from national data sources to get an indication of what is happening in rural America.

We have also selected these three areas because they represent services that are needed by major segments of the rural population and represent significant public health problems for all communities. As a result of government attention in the last several decades, elaborate categorical programs, reimbursement systems, and regulatory structures have grown up around each of these topics. The presence of these services in a rural community has an immediate and marked impact on the ability of inhabitants to obtain basic help—to maintain adequate oral hygiene and find relief from sudden dental pain, to have a means to cope with the unavoidable ravages of alcoholism and mental illness that exist in every community, and to care for the sick and the aged when they are no longer able to sustain an independent existence. The absence of these services impairs the community's ability to maintain its independence and homeostasis, forces people to travel to satisfy basic needs, and, in the case of long-term care, tends to break up and disperse families, forcing elderly people out of the towns where they have lived their lives.

It is beyond the scope of this book to discuss the contribution of the many ancillary health disciplines to rural health care. These include pharmaceutical services, podiatric care, physical therapy, occupational therapy, as well as a multitude of others. In addition to these components of the basic medical model, there are numerous non-traditional therapies and practitioners. Rural areas often are amply supplied with chiropractors, lay midwives, herbalists, and naturopaths, and their continued existence is testimony to the faith that rural dwellers place in their capabilities. Almost no research has been done that describes or evaluates their contributions to rural health care.

There is a need for additional research on the distribution, structure, and quality of services in the three topics we have selected as they are provided in rural areas. The majority of the articles and books written tend to be anecdotal collections of one-of-a-kind demonstration projects that may have great promise but have not been widely replicated. National statistics are sparse with regard to the urban and rural distribution of these services. Despite these limitations, we have tried to give a flavor of the way in which rural communities obtain these services and the problems that we perceive to be involved with assuring adequate distribution of care for the elderly and mental health and dental services in rural America.

HEALTH CARE FOR THE ELDERLY IN RURAL AMERICA

The proportion of elderly in the American population is rapidly increasing. In 1900, only 4.1 percent of the population were over 65 years of age; by 1975, the proportion of the population in this category had grown to 10.5 percent, a growth in numbers from 3.1 million to 22.4 million people.[1] This shift in the population pyramid of the United States will continue into the next millennium and will have a profound impact on the composition and functioning of our entire society.

Older people have a greater burden of chronic disease and use more of most kinds of health services than the population at large. The elderly use 4,100 days of hospital care annually for every 1,000 members of the population over 65 years old, a rate of utilization over four times that experienced by the population in general.[2] In addition, five percent of the entire elderly population live in a variety of long-term care institutions. The very old—those over 75 years of age—are the fastest growing segment of the aging population and require the most intensive assistance. The aging of the United States population will lead inexorably to higher demands for health services in the coming decades.

The rural aged have certain characteristics that distinguish them from the elderly population in general. As we discussed in Chapter 3, rural areas have larger proportions of elderly, with the highest concentrations of elderly—13 percent—found in totally nonmetropolitan counties.[1] Nine million of the 22.4 million elderly Americans live outside of urban areas and, as a result, tend to be further removed from the spectrum of social services for the aged that have sprung up across the country in the last decade.[3] The rural aged on the average are younger, more likely to be married, and less educated than elderly people living in urban areas.[4] In a review of the demographic data about the rural elderly, Youmans concludes that, "the rural aged, compared with urban older people, have substantially smaller incomes, are restricted in mobility because of inadequate transportation facilities, report poorer physical health, and reveal a more negative outlook on live."[5] Other studies have corroborated the finding that the rural elderly are in poorer general health even after correcting for the effects of age, sex, race, and poverty.[1]

Although the rural elderly have some distinct demographic characteristics, their use of health services does not differ markedly from the elderly population at large. Despite poorer health status, they use slightly fewer hospital days per year than the urban elderly;[2] their use of institutional long-term care services such as nursing homes is very similar to that of the urban aged; and differences in the rate at which old people are institutionalized has little to do with place of residence by itself.[6] Ninety-one percent of rural elderly were enrolled in Part B of Medicare, that portion of the program that covers physicians' services. Although there is virtually no difference between the rural and urban elderly in the proportion enrolled, users in metropolitan areas incurred significantly higher per-capita yearly charges.[7] This lower level of reimbursement, and a lower level of acute medical care utilization in general, reflect the relative lack of health services in rural areas and the lower fee structures that exist where those services are available.

The major differences between the rural and urban elderly seem to revolve more around living situations than health status. Rural elderly are more likely to be poorer and live in substandard housing, factors by themselves that would appear to have unfavorable consequences for health status. These negative attributes are counterbalanced, however, by the greater proportion of the rural elderly who are still living with spouses and belong to functioning social networks in the communities where they live. Several studies of rural elderly populations have shown that despite the apparently objective disadvantages of rural living, elderly people in rural areas felt that they could continue to live adequately in their home communities.[3,8] A review of the literature leads to the conclusion that the rural elderly are reticent to use existing services, even when they need them, either because they do not perceive the need or cultural attitudes cause a generalized reluctance to request assistance.[9]

From a review of the demographic data about the rural elderly, it is clear that there are subpopulations who are at extremely high risk. The rural aged who live alone are particularly susceptible to physical and social isolation. The almost total lack of organized transportation services in rural areas is a recurrent theme in all the discussions of this particular population segment and may have more pernicious consequences than the lack of specific services themselves.

THE PROLIFERATION OF SERVICES FOR THE AGED

The growing proportion of elderly in our society has been paralleled by a proliferation of social and health service programs designed for this demographic group. A review of the almost overwhelming number of programs that have evolved suggests that the number of programs has in fact outpaced the growth in the population they were designed to serve. Table 7.1 is a condensed list of the types of services that are currently available to the elderly, although all are not available in rural areas. There are endless variations on each of the services described in the table, and in many cases a categorical program with attending legislation, funding, and organizational structure has sprung up in response to a specific need.

One fundamental source of the proliferation of programs for the aged is the underlying diversity of the group itself. A recently retired, married, healthy 65-year-old carpenter does not need the same sort of assistance as that required by a debilitated, incontinent 87-year-old widow living in a nursing home. A taxonomy of aging has developed that separates the elderly into subgroups depending on their age, ranging from the "young-old" in their fifth and sixth decades of life to the "old-old" in their eighties and nineties.[10] When the divergent phases of aging are combined with extremely broad differences among the elderly in terms of health status and socioeconomic condition, one begins to understand the stimulus behind the wide and growing spectrum of services for the elderly. The difficulty, of course, for the rural areas is that the sparse population base cannot support or justify the multiple gradations of care. Although it is theoretically desirable to tailor each program to the individual needs of the recipient, rural areas must attempt to consolidate programs into multipurpose packages that can serve the broadest possible population.

Two major goals should underlie all the programs for the el-

TABLE 7.1. Spectrum of Services for the Elderly, United States, 1980

Institutional	Community-Based	In-Home
State mental hospitals	Geriatric day rehabilitation units	Visiting nurse
Acute care general hospitals	Day care	Homemakers
Chronic care hospitals	Sheltered workshops	Home health aides
Rehabilitation hospitals	Congregate meals	Chore services
Nursing homes	Community mental health centers	Meals on wheels
Skilled nursing facility	Senior Citizen centers	
Intermediate care facility	Geriatric ambulatory medical care	
Organized housing for the elderly	Legal services	
Group homes	Protective services	
Personal care homes		
Domiciliary care homes		
Foster homes		
Boarding houses		
Congregate care homes		
Retirement villages		
Hospices		
Respite care		

Source: Brody SJ, Masciocchi C: Data for long-term care planning by health systems agencies. *American Journal of Public Health* 70:1194–1198, 1980.

derly: retaining optimal level of functioning and maintaining social autonomy. Aging is a process of gradual functional deterioration; the objective of services for the aged is to retard that deterioration and enable the person with selected functional disabilities to maintain social and personal independence. The success of the social and health services directed to elderly populations is the degree to which they are able to live free, independent, and fulfilling lives. The wide spectrum of ambulatory services detailed in the second and third columns of Table 7.1 reflect society's commitment to preventing the premature institutionalization of the aged. Another strong financial motivation has been the explosive escalation in the costs of institutionalization, both in acute and chronic care facilities. To the degree that home health care and community services are less costly than institutional care, there are doubly strong motives for maintaining elderly people in their own homes.

Unfortunately, there is no coherent structure for planning, implementing, or administering services for the aged. Official responsibility for planning in this area has been divided among the Health Services Agencies (HSAs), the Area Agencies on Aging created by the Older Americans Act, community mental health centers, state public health institutions, and welfare agencies.[11] In addition, Medicare and Medicaid at both the federal and state levels have a tremendous stake and considerable influence over the nature and amount of services that are delivered because of their control of the bulk of financing for health care for the aged.[12] Other categorical programs, such as hospice care, arise in communities as the product of the work of voluntary agencies or concerned citizen's groups. There is no overall structure within which the various programs are logically placed.

THE NURSING HOME DILEMMA

"In the United States today, the nursing home has become the symbol of the inadequacy of the health system to meet the needs of the elderly."[13] This sweeping statement by Kane and Kane summarizes the sentiment and the frustration felt by many who have watched nursing homes become a multibillion dollar industry in the last decade, an industry that has threatened to bankrupt state treasuries and has unbalanced the entire Medicaid system. The frustration is heightened by the perception that, despite the drain on the private and public purse, many nursing homes are barely tolerable from both a medical and social perspective. Although the problem of nursing homes is a national one, an understanding of their place in our health system is important to this discussion of rural health care.

The nursing home, despite a poor overall reputation as the repository of the neglected, can play an important rule in maintaining community integrity. Although only five percent of the elderly population at any one time are in a long-term care facility, between 20 and 30 percent of the population will at some point during their lives live in a nursing home. The nursing home setting can be an important transitional placement for someone not needing the intensive care of a hospital setting but not yet ready to return home. For the rural community, access to local nursing home beds is essential to maintaining family integrity; in areas where nursing home beds are filled or unavailable, family members may be forced to move out of the communities where they have lived their lives.

The supply of nursing home beds varies from place to place. As Table 7.2 demonstrates, there is a marked regional discrepancy in the supply of nursing home beds. The supply of beds ranges from a high of 118.5 beds per thousand in Nebraska to 23.9 beds per thousand in Florida. The extreme discrepancies reflect a pervasive maldistribution in nursing home beds, a pattern perpetuated by historical accident and political power. Many rural areas are entirely without nursing home beds.

The supply of nursing home beds has expanded rapidly during the decade since the enactment of Medicare and Medicaid, with a 14 percent increase in beds during the period from 1971 to 1976 alone. Much more dramatic than the increase in the number of beds or the number of nursing home patients has been the explosion in costs. Table 7.3 summarizes the way in which Medicare and Medicaid funds have been expended in the decade between 1967 and 1977. Total Medicare expenditures increased 576 percent to over 18 billion dollars; Medicaid increased by over 700 percent to more than 16 billion dollars. Although the proportion of Medicare funds expended on nursing homes showed a small decrease during the decade, this decrease was more than counterbalanced by the increases in Medicaid nursing home expenditures.

TABLE 7.2. Nursing Home Beds per 1,000 Resident Population 65 Years of Age and Over, by Region for the United States

Geographic Region	Nursing Home Beds per 1,000 Residents 1971	Nursing Home Beds per 1,000 Residents 1976
New England	73.3	61.7
Middle Atlantic	42.8	47.1
East North Central	62.2	74.5
West North Central	81.1	83.2
South Atlantic	40.5	40.8
East South Central	41.0	47.2
West South Central	67.3	77.4
Mountain	56.9	57.0
Pacific	79.1	67.0
United States	58.6	61.7

Source: *Health, United States 1979.* USDHEW, PHS. DHEW Pub. No. (PHS) 80–1232, 1980, Table 63.

Figure 7.1 graphically presents the escalation in nursing home costs for the Medicaid population, an escalation that has showed no signs of slowing. The current monthly charge for nursing homes averages $689 per patient as compared to $186 in 1964.

This pattern is not a byproduct of a planned increase in services for the elderly population or the increase in the number of elderly in our population. Rather, it is the product—largely unforeseen—of the introduction of the Medicare and Medicaid programs and the impact of their reimbursement policies on long-term care. Medicare implemented a rigid classification system for nursing homes based on the amount of skilled nursing care provided.[14] Although this classification system is not entirely sensitive to patient medical needs and quite insensitive to their social needs or the overall health of the community, nursing homes have been forced to conform in order to receive reimbursement. The highest level of care is the Skilled Nursing Facility (SNF). Medicare will pay for care of patients in SNFs if they have been recently discharged from an acute care hospital and have a reasonable prospect of returning to their original home situation. However, the SNF classification is quite stringent, and there has been a decrease in the number of patients cared for in this environment. Intermediate Care Facilities (ICFs) are eligible for

TABLE 7.3. Percent Distribution of Medicare and Medicaid Expenditures, According to Type of Service, United States

Type of Service	1967		1977	
	Medicare[1] (percent)	Medicaid (percent)	Medicare[1] (percent)	Medicaid (percent)
Hospital care	76.0	40.2	74.0	31.5
Physicians' services	20.3	9.9	21.7	9.2
Nursing homes	3.1	33.7	1.9	39.2
Other services	0.7	16.2	2.3	20.1
Total expenditures (in millions)	$3,172	$2,271	$18,282	$16,300

Source: *Health, United States, 1979.* USDHEW, PHS, DHEW Pub. No. (PHS) 80–1232, 1980, Tables 79 and 80.
[1]Medicare recipients over 65 years of age.

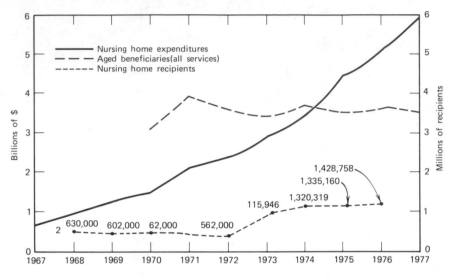

Figure 7.1. Medicaid and public assistance nursing home expenditures 1967–77, Medicaid aged beneficiaries 1970–77, and recipients 1968–75. (Health Care Financing Review, Winter 1980. DHEW Publication No. (HCFA) 03027-3/80.)

Medicaid reimbursement and constitute the category of nursing home that has grown most dramatically. Requiring less intense nursing care, patients in these settings tend to be those for whom the nursing home will be their last home before death. The patient in the ICF is very old, with an average age of 85;[15] these patients are likely to be frail, bedfast, widowed, and incontinent.[2]

The result of this reimbursement structure has been to create the nursing home industry as we know it today. As Table 7.4 shows, the majority of nursing homes are small, proprietary, intermediate care facilities. The nursing home industry has become an entrepreneurial endeavor, fueled by Medicaid dollars, staffed by poorly paid, minimally trained aides, and populated by elderly people no longer able to subsist in their homes. Typically, the SNFs are occupied by people with insurance or some personal resources; when their financial resources are depleted by the high costs of SNF care, they are moved to ICFs and become wards of the state.[16] Many states have also closed their chronic care hospitals and mental institutions. The result is that patients have been put in nursing homes, with the federal government subsidizing a major portion of the cost. The

TABLE 7.4. Number and Percent Distribution of Nursing Homes, Beds, and Residents by Selected Nursing Home Characteristics: United States, 1977

Nursing Home Characteristic	Nursing Homes		Beds		Residents	
	Number	Percent	Number	Percent	Number	Percent
ALL NURSING HOMES	18,900	100.0	1,402,400	100.0	1,303,100	100.0
Ownership						
Proprietary	14,500	76.8	971,200	69.3	888,800	68.2
Voluntary nonprofit	3,400	17.7	295,600	21.1	281,800	21.6
Government	1,000	5.5	135,700	9.7	132,500	10.2
Certification						
Skilled nursing facility only (SNF)	3,600	19.2	294,000	21.0	269,600	20.7
Medicare and Medicaid	2,100	11.3	204,500	14.6	190,300	14.6
Medicare	700	3.7	27,000	1.9	17,800	1.4
Medicaid	800	4.2	62,600	4.5	61,500	4.7
Skilled nursing facility and intermediate care facility (ICF)	4,600	24.2	549,400	39.2	527,800	40.5
Medicare SNF and Medicaid SNF and ICF	2,300	12.3	319,500	22.8	303,700	23.3
Medicaid SNF and ICF	2,100	10.8	218,700	15.6	213,800	16.4
Medicare SNF and Medicaid ICF	200	1.1	11,300	.8	10,300	.8
Intermediate care facility only	6,000	31.6	391,600	27.9	368,200	28.3
Not certified	4,700	25.0	167,400	11.9	137,500	10.6
Bed size						
Less than 50 beds	8,000	42.3	182,900	13.0	167,900	12.9
50–99 beds	5,800	30.8	417,800	29.8	397,000	30.5
100–199 beds	4,200	22.3	546,400	39.0	505,200	38.8
200 beds or more	900	4.6	255,400	18.2	233,000	17.9

Source: The National Nursing Home Survey: 1977 Survey for the U.S. USDHEW, National Center for Health Statistics, DHEW Pub. No. (PHS) 79–1794, June 1980.

problem thus created is that the nursing home becomes the last refuge for the mentally ill and the physically disabled.

We have painted a bleak picture of the nursing home, but the nursing home patient is not the only casualty. Because the costs of nursing homes have engulfed such large portions of state and federal budgets, there is a relative inability to fund other health and social service programs. Because nursing home costs are largely uncontrollable, legislators are forced to save in every other area. The United States spends far less on social services for the ambulatory elderly than almost every other industrialized country.[13] One of the reasons is that the Medicare and Medicaid programs were built in isolation with little consideration of their place within the entire health care delivery system. Although maintaining people in their home environments may not ultimately be less expensive than institutionalization, we currently have a system where we are not ever likely to know.[15]

INNOVATIONS IN CARE FOR THE RURAL ELDERLY

Although the problems of delivering adequate and appropriate health services to the elderly are massive, a number of innovative approaches have been attempted in rural areas. There are two common denominators to all these efforts. The first is trying to use an existing structure, service, or provider as the foundation for the service. The second is attempting to forge linkages between programs so that there is coordination instead of duplication at the local level. As a starting point, it is essential to consider health service as one on a spectrum of desirable social services rather than an isolated objective unrelated to housing, social interaction. or nutrition.

One of the most promising experiments in rural areas has been the use of underutilized beds in acute care hospitals for nursing home patients. Termed *swing-beds,* this approach offers hope of strengthening the financial base of the rural hospital while preserving and expanding long-term care capacity in rural communities. Swing-beds allow hospitals to receive reimbursement from Medicaid and Medicare for long-term care patients without undermining the basis under which the hospitals are reimbursed for acute care.

Ironically, it was the advent of third-party payment, such as Medicare, that strikingly reduced the spectrum of long-term care offered by hospitals. Historically, hospitals provided care to patients who today are sent to nursing homes. As a cost-saving measure, Medicare established rules that precluded hospital reimbursement for patients not requiring hospital services and established mechanisms for support of long-term care patients that spawned free-standing nursing homes. Whereas previously many hospitals routinely provided long-term care, currently only 400 of the more than 7,000 hospitals still provide Medicare-certified Skilled Nursing Facilities.[17] While the impact was marginal in large urban institutions, the strict exclusion of long-term patients has deepened the problem of low occupancy and inefficient utilization that plague small rural hospitals.

We have discussed the swing-bed concept extensively in the previous chapter. This approach is an excellent example of consolidating and coordinating services for the elderly in a rural community, building upon the foundation of preexisting community structures.[18,19] Rural hospitals can also incorporate other services for the elderly into their current operations. An example of such role broadening is the Northwoods Hospital in Phelps, Wisconsin. This 18-bed facility has incrementally added a 36-bed nursing home unit, started a senior citizens center, and sponsored the building of senior housing adjacent to the hospital. In this retirement community, the hospital was able to tailor its service mix to the changing demography of its population and improve financial viability at the same time.[20]

As illustrated in the previous example, innovative programs often stem from existing sources of health care in rural communities. One major problem with providing care to the elderly in rural areas has been the paucity of health providers. Rural physicians often are inundated with acutely ill patients; nursing home visits and home visits to the elderly may fall so far down on their lists of priorities as to be done perfunctorily if at all. One response has been the development of geriatric nurse practitioners, nurses who receive special training in the care of the elderly.[21] These nurses can become involved in home health care through existing local agencies and in certain circumstances can take the place of the physicians in routine visits to nursing home residents.[22] Although reimbursement barriers

in some states prevent the optimal utilization of this resource, using nurses to extend health care to the home-bound and the institutionalized is a concept that should be initiated and encouraged in rural areas.

Another change agent in the rural community is the extension agent, part of the extension service maintained by the Department of Agriculture. Extension agents are often highly respected members of their communities and can act as catalysts to bring new services to rural areas. Extension agents have the capacity to draw on the land-grant colleges in the states that support them and often have the knowledge and interest to become involved in areas of health and community development, an activity encouraged during the late 1970s. An example of such an activity in the area of aging is the "adult sitter" program begun under the aegis of the extension agents in West Virginia. The extension agent in each county organizes and trains volunteers to act as home health visitors for isolated, home bound elderly in their rural communities. In addition, they have started a variety of programs aimed at getting the elderly out of their homes and engaged in activities with other members of the community.[23] The program has many laudable elements: It targets a special high-risk group, uses existing personnel and administrative machinery for the organizational framework, and increases the community's ability to take care of its own.

The extension agent is an example of tapping into an existing network to bring services to rural communities without being forced to duplicate cumbersome and expensive administrative frameworks. A similar solution has evolved in North Carolina where the statewide Area Health Education Centers (AHECs) program has extended its resources in a wide variety of ways to rural communities. One example that has relevance to this discussion is that of a rural SNF faced with loss of accreditation because it did not have an adequate patient activity program in place. The nursing home could not afford to hire a recreational therapist to develop and administer such a program, but the AHEC was able to lend the services of such an individual on a part-time basis and thus establish the required program.[24] The same lesson applies with regard to many of the specialized activities and personnel that outside agencies require of rural nursing homes and hospitals. By establishing the resource centrally and then parcelling it

out to participating rural institutions on an as-needed basis, costs can be kept low and program quality high.

SUMMARY

The aging of the American population, and the growing stream of people choosing to retire in rural areas, guarantees that providing health care and social services for the elderly will remain a major challenge for rural communities. In a culture that treats aging as a stigma and often relegates the elderly to institutions to live out their days safely separated from the rest of society, relatively few resources have been invested in maintaining the autonomy and functional independence of the aged. Efforts to date have concentrated largely on financing a limited number of services through Medicare and Medicaid, and the unrestrained costs of these efforts have siphoned off resources that could have been used to maintain older people in their homes and communities.

Any rational program for the elderly, be it in rural or urban areas, must have as its centerpiece the prevention of premature institutionalization and the preservation of the individual as a functional member of society.[25] Health services—physician visits, hospital and nursing home care—are a component of a broader spectrum of social support. The older person may have a selected physical or mental deficit that is incompatible with independent living. Targeted assistance may enable such individuals to compensate for this deficiency and continue to live in their home environments.

Rural areas cannot support a wide variety of individual categorical services, each with its own administrative structure and single-purpose staff. There needs to be some point at which assessment and coordination occurs, a clearinghouse for the types of assistance that are available. The rural hospital has the potential for expanding its role into provisions of services for the elderly. The swing-bed concept should be investigated thoroughly, not only because of its effects on the economic viability of the hospital, but because it sensitizes hospital administration and staff to the needs of an important segment of the rural population.

It is also imperative that those interested in care for the aged build their programs upon other existing local and regional resources. The use of the county extension agent, cooperative arrangements with regional hospitals, universities, and elements of state government, and existing activities of local physicians and nurses should be maximized. Everyone in the rural community has a stake in the success of these efforts; aging is not a disease, but an inevitability.

RURAL MENTAL HEALTH PROGRAMS

Mental illness is a catch-all category for a very dissimilar collection of problems. Mental health is difficult to define with statistical precision. The dividing lines between eccentricity, social deviance, and out-and-out psychosis are difficult to draw and tend to be products of ethnocentric views of how the world should be ordered and how people should behave. Rural areas tend to have broader tolerance for certain kinds of deviance, but regional and cultural variation is considerable.

The majority of mental health problems stem from reactions to the common psychosocial stresses of life itself. Emotional distress is a universal human experience. Adjusting to birth, death, marriage, divorce, are the sorts of developmental tasks that everyone must confront. The majority of mental health problems stem from these sources, and in most cases it is useful to turn to others for advice, consultation, and support. Many turn to friends or clergy; many turn to the health care system, either for assistance with the physical consequences of psychic turmoil and stress or directly for help in adjusting to the strains, dislocations, and disappointments of life.

A second category of mental problem can be seen as related to inappropriate, unacceptable, or destructive behavior. This category would include the wide variety of addictive behaviors, most commonly alcohol and drug abuse, but gambling and food also can be the centers of self-destructive behavior patterns. Alcoholism is one of the most common afflictions of our culture and a cause of tremendous suffering and death. Drug abuse is common in every social class and location, often as the result of originally well-intentioned prescriptions for temporary emotional disturbance or transient pain.

Suicidal behavior is an example of a form of self-destruction that frequently involves the health care system. Certain forms of sociopathic behavior link the mental health and the criminal system in an often uncomfortable alliance.

The last large component of mental health ills are the psychotic ailments, in which people suffer major impairments in their ability to perceive reality and are unable to behave in a way that is acceptable within their cultural milieu. Schizophrenia is a remarkably common disease, with many variations in its expressions. Manic-depressive illnesses and severe depression are also very prevalent. These illnesses may wax and wane, but they are similar to severe physical disabilities in their impact on individuals and society.

Mental health care has become a separate dimension of the health care system, with its own cadre of workers, organizational structures, grant and research funds, and objectives. As a result of rapid biomedical advances and tremendous progress made in the field of psychopharmacology, hope was raised that emotional ills would yield to scientific progress and could be addressed by targeted programs. The community mental health movement grew and flourished during the 1960s and 1970s. Categorical federal funds were channeled to the field of mental health through the Community Mental Health Centers Act, which sponsored a nationwide network of centers designed to make mental health care available to all.[26]

It is important to note at the outset that the Community Mental Health Centers (CMHCs) and the community mental health movement that spawned them have not fulfilled the ambitious dreams of their originators. In fact, as this book is being written, there is a high likelihood that the entire community mental health center apparatus will be disassembled due to a lack of funding and enthusiasm by federal and state legislators. In reviewing the impact that CMHCs have had on the population at large, it is impossible to demonstrate that they have been able to make a significant contribution to the overall level of functioning of the population. Part of this is due to the difficulty we have in defining what constitutes good mental health; part of this is due to the fact that social and economic forces have more impact on the individual than the most innovative post hoc counseling intervention; and part of this is due to some underlying flaws in both the theory and practice that underlie the community mental health center movement.

As mentioned previously, there is little information available about the relative mental health status of rural dwellers. In a review of the literature, Flax summarizes, "In sum, although the accumulating evidence seems to support the notion that the mental health of rural areas is worse than that of urban, the conclusions are far from unambiguous."[27] Apparent differences seem to be more the consequence of the relative socioeconomic disadvantage of rural areas and a basically urban standard for measuring behavior rather than any underlying psychopathology attributable to rurality. It is clear that there are fewer mental health professionals in rural areas; only three percent of the nation's psychiatrists practice in rural America, and mental health professionals in general have a very strong tendency to locate in urban centers. Although the law establishing community mental health centers mandates rural services, only 13 percent of the funded centers claim to serve people in primarily rural catchment areas.[26] Those centers that do serve rural areas are more poorly staffed, offer fewer services, cover greater geographic areas, and are judged to be more deficient. In a federally sponsored review of all the CMHCs only 17.5 percent of the rural centers were felt to be structurally adequate.[28] Given the decrease in projected funding for existing centers and the decreasing inclination of U.S. medical graduates to choose psychiatry as a discipline, it is predictable that rural mental health services will become more scarce in the decade ahead.

THE RURAL COMMUNITY MENTAL HEALTH CENTER—LACK OF FIT

The challenge of the mental health care movement in the coming decade is to salvage something from the current structure of mental health centers before they cease to exist. The central conclusion in the literature is that the community mental health center is an urban creation that may have utility in the social service mix of the inner city but does not fit the medical needs or the social structure of the rural community. However, we have learned something from the experiences of the last 20 years, and it is important to use that knowledge as we plan for the future.

The CMHCs are required by law to provide a spectrum of essential services, including outpatient counseling services, inpatient psychiatric services, community consultation and education, partial hospitalization programs, such as day care, and emergency mental health services. Although most CMHCs provide a range of mental health interventions, their utilization is limited by small staffs, meager budgets, and a relatively low level of community acceptance.[29] The overwhelming tendency of rural CMHCs is to concentrate their time and energies on providing outpatient counseling services, although some creative attempts to use less conventional means of mental health care have occurred.

The major barrier to the success of CMHCs in rural areas is that the basic structure of rural communities is antithetical to the community mental health ethic. As Berry and Davis point out in a comprehensive review of the topic, the model that is espoused was designed by urban mental health workers for urban populations, but "clinics located in rural areas have problems that differ from those in urban centers . . . social factors peculiar to the rural area have not been taken into account."[30] The therapist, whether psychiatrist, nurse, or social worker, is alien to the rural community system, both because this professional is for the most part the product of an urban setting and educational system and because the rural community is a fishbowl in which people are reluctant to proclaim their deviance by visiting a mental health center. The rural ethic is basically conservative and stresses independence and stolid self-sufficiency; the mental health center forces the person to label himself or herself as outside the community standard by the act of seeking care. When care is sought, confidentiality is almost impossible to protect.

The result is that rural people are reluctant to use mental health services, even when they are ample and of high quality. In a study of the rural population in a southern county that had a functioning mental health clinic, "very few people considered the mental health clinic as a resource . . . even when the problem was clearly emotional. Our survey suggests that lack of knowledge about what constitutes mental health problems, typically associated with pejorative attitudes about such problems, is a major barrier to obtaining services."[31] In this study, and in most of the other work done on this subject, people consult their primary physician when confronted with a mental health problem, even when they recognize that emotional problems are the source of their difficulty and professional mental health workers are available. Consulting the physician carries none of the stigma of visiting a mental health center and allows the client to build upon an existing and comfortable relationship.

In addition to these cultural and psychological barriers, rural mental health centers are handicapped by other structural difficulties. Transportation, that common bugaboo of all centralized rural service programs, restricts access in particular to activities such as ongoing counseling that require frequent periodic attendance. Rural mental health centers have difficulty in reaching or caring for the long-term mentally ill client. Recruitment and retention of professional staff are particularly difficult in the mental health field, if only because of the inherent skepticism with which both rural patients and physicians frequently greet those trained in the somewhat ill-defined professions of mental health counseling and administration.[32] Studies of mental health workers who attempt to make the transition from urban to rural settings testify to the immense difficulties encountered. Rural settings require professionals to adopt the style and the language of the indigenous culture and leave behind the comfortable jargon of their field. Professional isolation is common, and faced with hostility and rejection, a high number drop out from the ranks.[33]

It is unnecessary to belabor the topic. The conventional model of the CMHC has not been successfully incorporated into rural communities. There appears to be little rationale for creating a system that provides mental health care that is separate from but parallel to the traditional health care system. However, it is possible to increase the capacity of the primary medical care system to recognize and appropriately treat mental health problems.

INTEGRATING MENTAL HEALTH SERVICES INTO TRADITIONAL MEDICAL CARE

Most mental health disorders can be divided into those that can be handled by the traditional medical system, those that require specialized attention from psychiatrists and other psychiatrically trained individuals, and those that require coordinated social service programs and support on a chronic basis. The problems of adjustment are best dealt with on an ambulatory basis within the normal support structure of the community, both lay and professional. Occasionally, specialized psychiatric consultation is required, but it is infeasible both from the standpoint of expense and the almost universal distribution of adjustment problems. Behavioral disorders require counseling assistance and an ability to manipulate the environment. Treatment may involve hospitalization, incarceration, behavioral therapy, or in some cases drugs, such as antabuse. Professional support is usually required. Psychotic patients tend to fall almost exclusively into the realm of the mental health professional. Where previously these patients were almost inevitably consigned to dreary state-supported psychiatric facilities, potent antipsychotic drugs have allowed these people to subsist in the community. Unfortunately, adequate community facilities often do not exist to help them maintain their medications and adjustment to the world, and the CMHCs have not been able to replace the mental hospital network.

In a survey of rural physicians, the practitioners indicate that the major psychiatric topics that they wished to learn more about centered around common diagnoses like depression and the use of short-term psychotherapeutic agents.[34] They were not interested in psychotic illness or long-term psychotherapy, which fall more into the domain of psychiatrists. They were uninvolved with the long-term residential programs that are the main form of support for the chronically mentally ill. There has been an increasing perception by a wide variety of observers that there must be an integration of basic health, mental health, and social service programs and that "problems in living" are best left to the primary health care provider.[35]

Some attempts have been made to formally merge programs involved with the delivery of primary care with those responsible for mental health care services. The Bureau of Community Health Services (BCHS)—sponsor of the Rural Health Initiative program described in Chapter 4—has attempted to encourage linkage of its rural programs with CMHCs operating in the same catchment areas. In 1977, BCHS and the National Institute of Mental Health entered into a formal agreement to stimulate rural cooperation and funded 57 rural projects to enable them to incorporate mental health professionals into ongoing primary health care delivery projects.[36] Although there have been some difficulties in actually incorporating these liaison personnel into the lives of the rural projects, the experiment has been promising. It is likely, unfortunately, that both programs will be casualties of the austerity of the 1980s. The underlying notion that the functions be combined is a sound one, however.

Part of the resistance to such efforts stems from the territorial imperatives that characterize many categorical programs. In a paper on rural mental health services, Hagebak illustrates the problem by citing as an example 114 separate federal programs, all of which fund transportation as part of their service package—yet it is very difficult to set up cooperative transportation systems among programs. He demonstrates that service integration, despite its unassailable logic, is a fragile concept and concludes that, "Any coordination or integration of rural human service must come from the professionals themselves—voluntarily, and in limited incremental steps."[37] Perhaps under the stimulus of wholesale dismantling of entire programs, self-interested cooperation will occur.

One tactic that has been quite successful in rural areas has been to develop mental health workers among volunteer staff made up of local individuals. In one rural county in Iowa, people recognized as natural helpers by virtue of their occupation or leadership roles in the community were recruited to take a series of training sessions to augment their natural talents. Using an educational model of intervention—a very useful and intuitively compelling approach— these people were trained to give a fairly full range of counseling services. The idea seemed to be popular both among the volunteers and the townspeople and had the twin virtues of using local individuals without incurring additional expense or building cultural barriers to care. [38]

Programs such as these that make use of the existing social structures that exist in all communities are a natural complement to augmenting the capability of the traditional health care system. In both cases, the rationale is to build additional services upon existing knowledge, organizational frameworks, and culturally enshrined patterns of trust. These methods are ideally suited to dealing with the first category of mental disruption, the ambulatory treatment of adjustment difficulties and emotional crises. However, it is also possible to increase the capacity of the rural health care system to deal with the more seriously disturbed mental patient in both the outpatient and inpatient setting.

A number of reports in the literature describe the initiation and implementation of inpatient psychiatric units in traditional rural acute general hospitals. In one such program in West Virginia, a psychiatrist affiliated with a CMHC used an incremental approach to introduce inpatient psychiatric services. Starting with a consultation service for local physicians, his first entry into the hospital field was to embark on a day-care program for selected patients. Building on the trust accumulated in this setting, he began to hospitalize selected nonthreatening patients in the regular acute care wards. The presence of these programs increased community demand among both patients and physicians for a fuller range of psychiatric services, and, ultimately, a separate psychiatric ward was established. Although this case is not typical—most rural hospitals are not as large as the one described here, nor are they able to attract skillful and highly motivated psychiatrists—it does illustrate that psychiatric patients can be taken care of in rural general hospitals. In the case mentioned here, the introduction of a local inpatient psychiatric resource nearly halved the number of patients requiring hospitalization at the state's chronic psychiatric hospitals.[39]

A more easily replicable example is reported in which local physicians maintained medical supervision of psychiatric patients admitted to a general rural hospital, and a group of psychiatrists assisted them from a distance through continuing consultation. The end results were similar to the previous case, with a greater proportion of the psychiatric inpatient needs met in the local area.[40] By increasing the scope of services offered by the rural hospital, one also bolsters the overall efficiency and long-term economic viability of the institution by using beds that would otherwise remain unfilled.

The future of mental health services in the rural areas will depend upon expanding the role of the local health care providers. A limiting factor in some rural areas will be the lack of primary care physicians. To the extent that organized mental health centers and mental health professionals remain available in rural areas, their focus should be on training, supporting, and encouraging the local system, rather than on providing direct patient care. The concerned community psychiatrist can have an enormous impact by ministering to the system of care, acting as a resource for the physician with a threatening or difficult patient, and maintaining the overall appropriateness and humanness of the services offered. Mental health and physical health are not divisible. The rural health care system must be built on this unity.

DENTAL CARE IN RURAL AMERICA

There are major differences between the fields of medicine and dentistry that have important implications for rural health care. Although both physicians and dentists spend four years in professional schools, the majority of physicians spend an additional three years in residency training after graduation from medical school. Dentists rarely take residencies, and the majority of all dentists remain in private general practice. More importantly, physicians—particularly those now emerging from training—practice in group settings, sharing economic and professional concerns with their partners. Dentists have traditionally been independent entrepreneurs, practicing alone, although in urban areas more recent dental graduates are joining group practices. By the nature of their work, physicians spend a considerable portion of their time in formal institutional settings, such as hospitals and nursing homes. In these settings, their work is under constant scrutiny, and the content of their practice is constrained by regulation, supervision, and tradition. Dentists control the style and content of their practice life, constrained primarily by market forces, as well as professional norms.

The dental profession also differs from the medical profession in other important aspects. The bulk of medical costs are covered by third-party insurance plans. By contrast, although there has been an increase in the amount of dental insurance in force, the majority of dental care is paid for out of pocket by the consumer.[41] Patient demand for dental care is quite sensitive to overall economic conditions and varies greatly from one region of the country to another. Dental care is generally perceived as an elective procedure by most consumers, and thus the value that people put on oral health has a direct effect on the overall demand for dental care.[42]

Another way in which the dental profession differs from the medical profession is the way in which licensing boards restrict the freedom of dentists to choose where they will practice. Dentists tend to be much more geographically restricted than physicians, and part of the reason is that dentists must, for the most part, take state board exams in every state where they wish to practice. Although ostensibly designed as a quality assurance technique, the effect of state dental boards is to exclude dentists from entering certain states, particularly those states that already have what local dentists perceive to be an ample supply of practitioners. Those states with high per-capita incomes are those states where dental incomes are high—and where a new dental applicant is more likely to fail the state board exam.[43,44]

From the standpoint of rural health care, the configuration of the dental profession is such that it is actually easier in many ways to sustain a dental practice in a rural area than a medical practice. One of the major constraints on the physician wishing to practice in a rural area is the burden of constant availability; the rural physician must arrange to provide continuous care for patients, and it is this 24-hour call responsibility that is frequently the limiting factor in the survival of a medical practice. In addition, the physician seeks access to hospital facilities, and only towns that have a certain minimum population base can afford to provide a hospital. Dentistry suffers from neither of these constraints. The dentist generally is under no obligation to provide assured 24-hour-a-day coverage; most dental procedures can be deferred, and even dental emergencies are more a matter of patient discomfort than any threat to life. Dentists also do not depend on hospitals for their economic survival and professional growth. Each dental office is self-sufficient, and dentists can hire as many or as few assistants or auxiliaries as needed to match the dental demand in the community where they practice.

On the other hand, the dentist as an entrepreneur is more a captive of the economic status of the community and the extent of effective consumer demand. An impoverished rural town where dental care is not highly valued makes poor soil in which to start a practice. The young dentist is less likely than the physician to find public assistance in starting a practice and typically has to finance privately the relatively expensive equipment required to set up a modern office. Unless the dentist has patience and persistence and a talent for marketing his or her services, he or she may not be able to build a rural practice fast enough to meet the amortization costs of the equipment purchased. Therefore, although a dentist may be professionally capable of sustaining an autonomous practice in a rural area, the uncertain economic rewards and unpredictable practice growth may dissuade him or her from accepting the challenge.

THE RURAL DENTIST REMAINS IN SHORT SUPPLY

There is a profound maldistribution of dentists in this country, a maldistribution that has yet to yield to the rapid expansion in the number of dental schools and dental graduates over the last 20 years. Table 7.5 shows the distribution of active civilian dentists per 100,000 population in the United States at the end of 1979. The data illustrate the effect of city size, population density, and socio-economic status on the distribution of dentists. Dentists distribute themselves along a population gradient, with few dentists in the most rural communities.[45] When this is added to marked regional variations in the supply of dentists, we see that areas of the country like the rural South have only about 35 percent as many dentists relative to the population as the urban Northeast. The differences are even more striking for the small rural towns of fewer than 5,000 people. For these communities, there are only 27 dentists per 100,000 population, half the national average, and some states have fewer than 15 dentists per 100,000 population.

Dentists' preferences for urban areas have contributed to an inadequate supply of dentists in rural America, and many rural communities have been designated as dental shortage areas by the federal government. As shown in Table 7.6, most of the 881 designated areas are in nonmetropolitan counties; in all, the government estimates that almost 20 million people live in areas where there are insufficient numbers of dentists and that it would require an additional 3,000 dentists to remedy the deficiency. In 1976, there were 267 counties that had no dentists at all and an additional 710 counties with fewer than one dentist for each 5,000 inhabitants; most of these counties were in rural areas.

The supply of dentists is closely related to the amount of dental care a population receives. Table 7.7 demonstrates that the same gradient that determines the supply of dentists also affects both the percentage of the population visiting a dentist within any given year and the average number of dental visits per year. Rural areas have the

TABLE 7.5. Ratio of Active Civilian Dentists to Population in Metropolitan and Nonmetropolitan Counties in the United States, December 31, 1979

		Active Civilian Dentists per 100,000 Population					
		Metropolitan Areas by Population			Nonmetropolitan Counties by Size of Central City		
Geographic Area	All Areas	Total	1,000,000 or More	Under 1,000,000	Total	10,000 or More	Under 10,000
North East	66	70	76	60	46	47	43
North Central	52	57	61	51	41	47	35
South	44	51	56	49	29	37	24
West	62	65	68	61	47	51	40
Total	54	60	66	54	37	44	31

Source: Health Resources Administration, Bureau of Health Professions, Division of Health Professions Analysis, November 14, 1980. Unpublished tabulations.

255

TABLE 7.6. Number of Dental Shortage Areas Designated in Metropolitan Areas and Nonmetropolitan Counties and Additional Dentists Needed in the United States, June 30, 1980

Geographic Area	Number of Dental Shortage Areas			Population of Designated Areas (in thousands)	Number of Dentists Needed
	Total	Metro	Nonmetro		
North East	66	32	34	2,503	382
North Central	192	28	164	3,918	664
South	496	72	424	10,315	1,507
West	103	23	80	1,651	287
Other areas	24	—	24	871	204
Total	881	155	726	19,258	3,044

Source: Health Resources Administration, Bureau of Health Professions, Division of Health Professions Analysis, November 14, 1980. Unpublished tabulations.

TABLE 7.7. Population to Dentist Ratios and Visits to Dentists by Geographic Region and Place of Residence.

	Population to Dentist Ratio, 1977	Percent of Population with Dental Visits During One Year	Average Number of Dental Visits Per Person per Year
Geographic Region			
North East	1,562	51.2	1.9
North Central	2,053	47.4	1.4
South	2,396	40.5	1.2
West	1,595	48.1	1.8
United States	1,905	46.3	1.5
Place of Residence			
Metropolitan areas	1,701	49.4	1.8
Nonmetropolitan areas			
Nonfarm	2,575	43.1	1.2
Rural	3,664	41.9	0.9

Source: Health Resources Administration, Bureau of Health Professions, Division of Health Professions Analysis, January 1977. Unpublished tabulations.

fewest dentists in relation to population size, and rural residents use the fewest dental services. As noted previously, the supply and demand of dental care are highly interrelated. Rural residents are unable to obtain services because of the unavailability of dentists, but their low rate of utilization also deters dentists from settling in these underserved areas.

The data for dental care are more stark than for medical care in general. There is a shortage of dentists and dental care in rural communities, with the smallest and poorest rural communities suffering the most acute deficiencies.

ATTEMPTS TO REMEDY RURAL DENTAL SHORTAGES

The major strategy used to improve the distribution of dentists in the United States has been to increase the number of dentists. The dentist-to-population ratio remained stable from 1920 to 1969, at which time the relative supply of dentists began to decline. In 1964, it was found that the overall supply of active civilian dentists was 44.8 per 100,000 population, down from the historical plateau of 49.9. A formal federal review of the situation in 1967 generated a report that predicted continuing decline unless steps were taken to increase the number of dental graduates.

In the late 1960s and 1970s, a series of health manpower legislative efforts was initiated, stimulating rapid expansion in the number of dentists in training. The number of accredited dental schools grew from 47 in 1962 to 60 in 1980, with much of the growth occurring in the South where the need was greatest. Capitation grants to dental schools also encouraged schools to increase their class sizes, and the number of graduates increased from 3,253 in 1960 to 5,150 in 1980, a 58.5 percent increase.[46]

At the same time, there was a concerted effort to increase the productivity of existing dentists. The approach chosen was to train a generation of dental auxiliaries—dental assistants, hygienists, dental laboratory technicians, and others—who would either assist the dentist in the labor-intensive process of giving dental care or actually take on the job of providing certain low-complexity dental services. The effect of this effort has been to create a very large labor supply of dental paraprofessionals and new streamlined techniques of dental treatment, which accompanied the significant expansion in the supply of dentists.[47]

These changes are reflected in the dentist supply figures presented in Table 7.8. Regional differences remain profound, but the overall supply relative to the population has grown 15 percent in the decade of the 1970s. Unfortunately, however, this increased supply of dental practitioners has not yet begun to have a significant impact on underserved rural areas.

Table 7.9 illustrates this rather frustrating state of affairs. From 1974 to 1979 there was an eight percent expansion in the relative supply of dentists, but these dentists for the most part have chosen to locate in those areas that already are well supplied. The largest gainers have been small cities and suburbs, those communities where the most dentists already practice. The inner-city portions of large metropolitan areas have gained few dentists and for communities with fewer than 5,000 people—the demographic category that accounts for the majority of rural towns—the relative increase in dental manpower was a negligible 3.5 percent. Even more discouraging is the fact that only 50 percent of the entire population visits dentists at least once a year, a figure that has remained static over the last decade for the population as a whole.

Other attempts to remedy the maldistribution problem have been meager and largely ineffective. In 1978, the American Association of Dental Schools passed a resolution asking the schools "To consider providing more dentists for rural communities and other areas of short supply."[48] In 1980, a follow-up questionnaire sent to the dental schools that had committed themselves to this endeavor revealed that essentially nothing had been done. The only program gaining some currency was the establishment of extramural preceptorships for dental students in the hope that this experience would introduce them to alternative places in which dentistry might be practiced. However, the overall conclusion of the study was "that most dental schools have not yet become actively involved in efforts to solve maldistribution problems."[48]

One program that has shown some limited promise has been the establishment of a placement network for dentists. The previous study revealed that there is very little coordination among dental schools, dental societies, and government agencies in inducing den-

TABLE 7.8. Number of Active Civilian Dentists and Dentist-to-Population Ratios, United States.

Geographic Area	1970		1975		1979	
	Active Dentists	Dentists per 100,000 Population	Active Dentists	Dentists per 100,000 Population	Active Dentists	Dentists per 100,000 Population
North East	28,601	59	31,983	65	32,418	66
North Central	26,129	46	28,146	49	30,137	52
South	22,025	35	25,255	38	30,795	44
West	18,925	55	21,356	57	24,980	62
Total	95,680	47	106,740	51	118,330	54

Source: Health Resources Administration, Bureau of Health Professions, Division of Health Professions Analysis, October 3, 1980. Unpublished tabulations.

TABLE 7.9. Percent Increase in Number of Active Civilian Dentists per 100,000 Population from 1974 to 1979 for Metropolitan and Nonmetropolitan Areas

	Dentists per 100,000 Population		Percent Increase
	1974	1979	
Metropolitan Areas	56	60	7.1
1,000,000 or more	62	66	6.1
Under 1,000,000	48	54	12.5
Nonmetropolitan Counties	34	37	8.8
Central city 25,000 or more	43	50	16.3
Central city 10,000 to 24,999	36	50	11.1
Central city 5,000 to 9,999	32	35	9.4
Central city under 5,000	26	27	3.5
United States	50	54	8.0

Source: Health Resources Administration, Bureau of Health Professions, Division of Health Professions Analysis, November 14, 1980. Unpublished tabulations.

tists to settle in places where they are really needed. One notable exception to this lack of coordination was a program started in Minnesota in 1972. In this instance, the dental profession and the state licensing board initiated a dental information service that made dental graduates aware of practice opportunities, particularly those in rural areas. The service has been widely used, and an increased proportion of graduating students have located in underserved rural areas during the period that the program has been operational.[49] Although one cannot unambiguously relate this outcome to the initiation of the information service, this is an example that may bear fruit of some cooperative efforts.

The Minnesota program has since been extended into a National Health Professions Placement Network funded by the Kellogg Foundation. This project is aimed primarily at dental groups and has as its aim "to facilitate the flow of dental manpower in response to the demands of the population."[50] It operates a computerized clearinghouse that puts dental graduates in touch with communities with expressed needs for dentists. As a voluntary effort sponsored by the dental profession, it has found wide acceptance within the profession.[51]

One direct attempt to remedy problems of dental maldistribution has been the National Health Service Corps (NHSC). The NHSC designates underserved communities as shortage areas and then—in concert with local nonprofit sponsoring organizations—recruits and places dentists in these areas. This approach has the advantage of simplicity. It is a direct intervention, rather than an indirect approach depending on the trickle-down effect of expanded class size. However, because it is viewed by the dental profession as federal interference in health care, the profession has been opposed to the program and quite successful in preventing its widespread implementation. Recent changes in federal health policy, if carried out, will mean the fairly rapid demise of the NHSC as an instrument of change in the field of dentistry and the end of this promising but thwarted approach.

WHAT THE FUTURE HOLDS

Dentistry is a profession in transition. As a recent article proclaimed, "Thus to say that the dental profession in the 1980's is in a turmoil is almost an understatement of our current situation. As a result of prognostications which are based on so many unknown factors, changes may take place which are irreversible or reversible at great expense to the community and could have permanent negative effects on the lives of individuals and on the population in general."[46] Underlying this rhetoric is the perception by dentists that their current economic stature may be beginning to erode. Dentists in the United States have been secure and well paid for their labors. However, they feel that the combination of increasing numbers of dental graduates, the profusion of auxiliaries, and a poorly growing economy threaten their current economic status. In some states, denturists and dental hygienists are assuming expanded functions and are being granted legal sanction to practice independently. In others, third-party payers are restricting fee schedules and subjecting proposed dental treatments to increased scrutiny. Widespread fluoridation has decreased the overall prevalence of caries. Dentists project an unsure future for themselves.

What impact will this have on rural America? Economic logic would suggest that as competition intensifies, dentists will migrate into rural areas where the markets are not so saturated and the need for dentists is greater. Although there is some anecdotal evidence to suggest that this may be beginning to happen, there are no statistical data that as yet corroborate this trend. Dentists appear to be very reluctant to leave urban areas, and licensing barriers further inhibit the free movement of dentists among states and regions. Further expansion of dental schools seems highly unlikely, and with the shrinking of the National Health Service Corps, the major direct intervention technique will disappear.

Thus the outlook for improved dental care in rural areas is not particularly hopeful. Dentistry as a profession has not been responsive to the needs of underserved rural populations, and state and federal interest in the issue is waning. Until the public decides that dental care is an important local service, little change can be expected.

REFERENCES

1. McCoy JL, Brown DL: Health status among low-income elderly persons: Rural-urban differences. *Social Security Bulletin*, June 1978. Report No. 4 from the Survey of Low-Income Aged and Disabled. DHEW Pub. No. (SSA) 78–11700.
2. Kovar MG: Health of the elderly and use of health services. *Public Health Reports* 92:9–19, 1977.
3. Costello TP, Pugh RC, Steadman BF, et al: Perceptions of urban versus rural hospital patients about return to their communities.
4. Nelson G: Social services to the urban and rural aged: The experience of area agencies on aging. *Gerontologist* 20:200–207, 1980.
5. Youmans EG: The rural aged. Annals of the American Academy of Political and Social Sciences 429:81–90, 1977.
6. McCoy JL, Edwards BE: Contextual and Demographic Antecedents of Institutionalization Among Aged Welfare Recipients. Paper presented at annual meeting of the American Statistical Association, August 11, 1980, Houston, Texas.

7. Supplementary Medical Insurance: *Utilization and Charges for the Aged, 1974.* Research and Statistics Notes, HCFA, June 1978. US Governmment Printing Office: 1978–261–684:1044.

8. Kivett VR, Learner RM: Perspectives on the childless rural elderly: A comparative analysis. *Gerontologist* 20:708–716, 1980.

9. Hayslip B, Ritter ML, Oltman RM, et al: Home care services and the rural elderly. *Gerontologist* 20:192–199, 1980.

10. Coward RT: Planning community services for the rural elderly: Implications from research. *Gerontologist* 19:275–282, 1979.

11. Brody SJ, Masciocchi C: Data for long-term care planning by health systems agencies. *American Journal of Public Health* 70:1194–1198, 1980.

12. Callahan JJ, Diamond LD, Giele JZ, et al: Responsibility of families for their severely disabled elders. *Health Care Financing Review* 1:29–48, 1980.

13. Kane RL, Kane RA: Care of the aged: Old problems in need of new solutions. *Science* 200:913–919, 1978.

14. Willemain TW, Bishop CE, Plough AL: *The nursing home "level of care" problem.* Monograph from University Health Policy Consortium, Brandeis University, Waltham, Massachusetts, February 1980.

15. Tobin SS: The mystique of deinstitutionalization. *Society* 15:73–75, July-August 1978.

16. Hadden BF, Cohen J: A new campaign of caring for the aged: Perspectives and prescriptions. *Journal of Health and Human Resources Administration* 3:148–168, 1980.

17. Miller DR, Rosenthall JM: Swing beds can work—With good planning. *Hospitals* 54:97–98, 100, 102–103, 1980.

18. Aland KM, Walter BA: Hospitals in Utah reduce còsts, improve use of facilities. *Hospitals* 52:85–87, 1978.

19. Shaughnessy P, Tynan EA, Landes D, et al: *An evaluation of swing bed experiments to provide long-term care in rural hospitals.* Denver, Colo, Center for Health Services Research, University of Colorado Health Sciences Center, March 1980.

20. Friedman E: Little hospital has big ideas. *Hospitals* 54:89–94, November 16, 1980.

21. Ham R: Alternatives to institutionalization. *American Family Physician* 22:95–100, 1980.

22. Williams GO: The elderly in family practice: An evaluation of the geriatric nurse practitioner. *Journal of Family Practice* 5:369–373, 1977.

23. Lohmann N, Dial W: The extension agent in the rural aging services

continuum, in Hoffman DH, Lamprey H (eds): *Rural Aging.* Lexington, Council on Aging, University of Kentucky, 1979.

24. Cozart ES, Evashwick C: Developing a recreational program for patients in a rural nursing home. *Public Health Reports* 93:369–374, 1978.

25. Levitan AB: Nursing home dilemma? Transfer trauma and the non-institutional option: A review of the literature. *Clearinghouse Review* 13:653–659, 1980.

26. Jones JD, Wagenfeld MO, Robin SS: A profile of the rural community mental health center. *Community Mental Health Journal* 12(2):176–181, 1976.

27. Flax JW, Ivens RE, Wagenfeld MO, et al: Mental health and rural America: An overview. *Community Mental Health Review* 3:1–15, 1978.

28. Hoagland M, Ozarin LD: *A new day in rural mental health services.* USDHEW, PHS, ADAHMA, NIMH, USGPO, Stock Number 017-024-00760-9, 1978.

29. Gertz B, Meider J, Pluckhan ML: A survey of rural community mental health needs and resources.

30. Berry B, Davis AE: Community mental health ideology: A problematic area for rural areas. *American Journal of Orthopsychiatry* 48:673–679, 1978.

31. Lee SH, Gianturco DT, Eisdorfer C: Community mental health center accessibility: A survey of the rural poor. *Archives of General Psychiatry* 31:335–339, 1974.

32. Cedar T, Salasin J: *Research Directions for Rural Mental Health.* McLean, Va, The Mitre Corporation, 1979.

33. Riggs RT, Kugel LF: Transition from urban to rural mental health practice. *Social Casework* 57:562–567, 1976.

34. Callen KE, David D: What medical students should know about psychiatry: The results of a survey of rural general practitioners. *American Journal of Psychiatry* 135:243–244, 1978.

35. Morrill RG: The future for mental health in primary health care programs. *American Journal of Psychiatry* 135:1351–1355, 1978.

36. Goldman HH, Burns BJ, Burke JD: Integrating primary health care and mental health services: A preliminary report. *Public Health Reports* 95:535–539, 1980.

37. Hagebak BR: Mental health services in rural areas: The case for intra-agency coordination and service integration. Paper presented at third annual Georgia Primary Health Care Conference, April 1980.

38. Kelley VR, Kelley PL, Gauron EF, et al: Training helpers in rural mental health delivery. *Social Work* 22:229–231, May 1977.

39. Ames DA: Developing a psychiatric inpatient service in a rural area. *Hospital and Community Psychiatry* 29:787–791, 1978.
40. Werner A, Knarr FA, Stack JM: Psychiatric services in a rural general hospital. *International Journal of Psychiatry in Medicine* 8(1):25–34, 1978.
41. Littleton PA: Dental manpower supply and requirements: The effect of national estimates on individual dental schools. *Journal of Dental Education* 44:241–245, 1980.
42. Born DO: Manpower distribution and costs. pp. 129–141.
43. Benham, L, Maurizi A, Reder MW: Migration, location and remuneration of medical personnel: Physicians and dentists. *Review of Economics and Statistics* 50:332–347, 1968.
44. Born DO: Dental manpower planning and distribution: A survey of the literature. *Advances in Socio-Dental Research* 2:5–26, 1975.
45. 1980 Report to the President and Congress on the Status of Health Professions.
46. Waldman HB, Pollack BR: Risks in forecasting in the health field. *Journal of the American College of Dentists* 47:149–163, 1980.
47. Do we really need more dentists? *Dental Management* 14:55–62, December 1974.
48. McDonald RE, Barton P: Activities by the schools to improve the distribution of dentists: An AADS report. *Journal of Dental Education* 44:246–247, 1980.
49. Born DO, Burton K: Impact of a computerized placement service on practice location of recent graduates. *Journal of the American Dental Association* 97:175–178, 1978.
50. Born DO: The national health professions: New hope for an old problem? *New Dentist* 28–30, 1979.
51. O'Neal V: ADA network helps dentists relocate. *Dental Economics* 54–56, June 1980.

CHAPTER 8

Toward a Strategy for Improving Rural Health Care

Rural America today bears little resemblance to the agrarian society that prevailed when this nation was founded. By the same token, rural health care services and the people who provide them are but distant cousins of their colonial forebears. These are not the best of times nor the worst of times for rural America. But they are rapidly changing, confusing, and often contradictory times.

The purpose of this chapter is to rise above the detail of the previous discussion. As this book is written, the New Deal concept of an assertive central government is being challenged by powerful political forces, and the fate of many major federal programs is in doubt. Even during this period of flux, general conclusions can be drawn about the future problems in health care that will confront rural communities. Potential solutions to these problems can be extracted from the enormous amount of experience that we have collected in providing health care in a wide variety of rural settings. Although there has been an ebb and flow in the amount of national attention to rural concerns, and a parallel rise and fall in the health services available in rural areas, certain basic axioms transcend these periodic currents.

These principles can be useful. Among the most distressing and disruptive characteristics of our political system as it affects the

267

status of rural health care are the wide, sudden swings in public policy and direction. Rural health concerns are whipsawed back and forth by abrupt shifts in philosophy, program structure, and changing social truisms. Those responsible for the design, implementation, and actual delivery of health services are buffeted by these changes and waste considerable energy reacting defensively to the latest threat. Only by formulating a clear set of objectives and having some useful principles to guide our course can we hope to make any long-term progress toward our goals.

This chapter sets out six general principles for the planning and delivery of rural health services. After setting out these principles, we will discuss them in relation to several major aspects of the rural health care delivery system to illustrate how they might be applied in actually improving rural health care services.

BASIC PRINCIPLES UNDERLYING AN EFFECTIVE RURAL HEALTH CARE SYSTEM

The giving and getting of health care does not occur in isolation. Patients and doctors, hospitals and nursing homes, medical schools and insurance companies are all part of a very complex enterprise that revolves around the provision of medical care. Although medical care in the United States comes in many different kinds of packages, it is still part of a system in that each part is interconnected. Changes in medical education policy have long-term implications for the type of physicians who practice in rural America. New diagnostic technologies exert pressure for change on rural hospitals. Modifications in health care financing affect the way in which people utilize health care.

The optimal provision of health care in the rural setting depends upon some understanding of the dynamics of this system. In most rural communities, decisions about health care are made by a broad segment of the population and include the medical professionals, local health administrators, public officials, and the informal power structure of the community. Citizens in general help shape the system with their votes on hospital levies, through their contributions to the local hospital, by participating in the volunteer ambulance service, and by deciding where they will go for their own health care.

All of these actors need some understanding of the fit between the rural health care system and the larger medical system of which it is a part. Although the best health planning is that which originates within the local community, local planning cannot occur in a vacuum. The principles described below all derive from the fundamental concept that rural health care must be integrated into the larger medical care system.

PLANNING MUST BE POPULATION BASED

Planning is in some way inimical to the American character. Health planning in particular has been an expensive and largely unlamented failure. Despite exponential increases in the cost of health care, serious and persistent inequities in the distribution of and access to health care, and increasing public dissatisfaction with the health care that is received, no effective national strategy has emerged. In fact, the largely symbolic planning edifices, such as Health Systems Agencies, are being systematically dismantled. They are being dismantled because they run counter to the politically prevailing ideology that invisible market forces will of themselves shape the system and because planning efforts to date have had little effect on medical care costs or the quality of the health care system.

The end of nationally mandated planning will have little impact on rural areas. National guidelines promulgated as part of the health planning laws have been almost ludicrously insensitive to rural concerns. The outpouring of rural outrage following the suggestion that rural hospitals close their obstetric services was so politically effective that large-scale rural exemptions were incorporated into the guidelines. In most cases, rural communities have found ways to circumvent any planning guidelines that would have significantly impaired their freedom to maneuver.

The unfortunate side effect of this dismal failure is that rural communities have in many cases concluded that planning is antithetical to their own interests. The real lesson of this experience is that planning needs to be locally initiated and controlled, and that health care plans should be based on the needs of the population to be served rather than some remote, irrelevant theoretical construct. Only by knowing the demographic structure of the target population

and the volume and type of medical and social services the population will require can rural communities build health institutions that
will meet those needs.

Planning is not an arcane science; it is the common sense process
of finding out what you need and what must be done to meet that
need. An unfortunate outgrowth of the planning laws has been the
creation of a professional guild of planners who have little actual
experience in providing or administering health services. Planning
should be done by the people who will bear the consequences of the
plan—the doctors and nurses, administrators, and future clients of
the newly developed system.

The process of developing a local plan for health services is
straightforward. *First,* the local community must define its medical
service area. Medical service areas do not in general follow convenient geopolitical boundaries like townships or counties; they tend to
mirror prevailing trade patterns for other major goods and services.
In defining the medical service area, the local planners must take into
account the distinction between those services that will be provided
within the area and those services for which people will have to
travel. This requires an understanding of the location and flow of
medical services within the larger region of which the rural community is a part. In general, a useful goal for planning is to make primary
care services—both inpatient and outpatient—available to people
without forcing them to spend too much time traveling. One-half
hour is the figure suggested in Chapter 6, but this must be modified
by considerations of local geography, weather, and the availability of
decent roads and public transportation.

Once the medical service area has been roughly defined, the
second step is to calculate the number of people living within the
service area and the age and sex structure of the population. Census
data, corrected by information from the utility and telephone companies, and various state and county data sources provide the raw
data for this task. Population trends must also be calculated so that at
least some approximation can be made of what the future holds in
terms of the number and type of people that will be needing health
services. A useful planning horizon is 10 years hence, and many of
the desirable changes that one would prescribe for a rural area could
take up to 10 years to bring about.

The *third* step is to estimate the total amount of medical services
that the population in the service area will use. This entails ap-

proximating the number of visits that will be made to physicians in their offices and the number of medical, surgical, and obstetric admissions to the hospital that can be expected to occur in this population during a one-year period. Exact figures for these rates may not be available for every small community, but a little ingenuity will allow reasonable approximations. Precise national data from the Health Interview Survey and the National Ambulatory Medical Care Survey allow one to determine the volume of medical services consumed by people in each stage of their lives. More refined data may be available within the state, county, local hospital, or doctor's office. In any case, it is possible to calculate with acceptable precision the total amount of health care that the target population will use—and therefore begin the process of deciding how and where to provide those services.

The *fourth* step is critical and controversial and has the most far-reaching implications—partitioning. Partitioning means deciding in advance whether the required medical care will be provided within the rural community or outside the target area. In order to reduce the conflict and make the process rational and defensible, partitioning should be done on a service by service basis. That is, for each type of hospital or ambulatory service that the rural population requires, a decision is made as to where it could be best supplied. The problem of determining the optimal location is not simple; there are no hard and fast guidelines. In general, the major determinants of the decision are quality, cost, and community acceptability.

The most important criterion must be quality: Can the indicated service be safely provided in the rural community, or would a local person be exposed to significantly less risk if he were to receive the service somewhere else? For some services the answer is obvious; no small rural hospital aspires to perform open-heart surgery. By the same token, virtually every rural community will seek to provide basic stabilization and transport of emergency victims. The difficult decisions will revolve around controversial items such as routine elective surgery and obstetric care. In these cases, it is useful to review the research findings—touched on in Chapter 6—which show the relationship between the frequency with which procedures are done or services rendered and the outcome of those interventions. In addition, it may be possible to review local experience and flag those services where quality has been deficient when compared to that available elsewhere.

The second standard is cost. The procedure may be relatively harmless but require such expensive equipment that the projected amount of use does not justify the investment. By the same token, certain services may depend upon specialized personnel who could be underused because of the insufficient demand for that activity within the medical service area. Since the community ultimately pays for all the services that it provides, some sort of cost screen is essential.

The third yardstick is community acceptability. Local custom, historical antecedents, and the current mix of physicians and administrators will have an effect on what solution is best fitted to the community in question. To be acceptable, any plan must proceed from current reality. A town with a young, vigorous, and well-accepted orthopedic surgeon will probably make some provision for orthopedic surgical procedures within the local hospital, even if there is a slightly higher cost associated with so equipping the operating suite. For the plan to work, it must recruit the support of the major decision makers in the area. A pristine, theoretically faultless plan is of no use if it molders on the shelf or disrupts the community.

The *fifth* step is to assemble the individual services into logically coherent packages and then determine the people, facilities, and financing necessary to deliver them. This package must take into account preexisting services and people in the rural community. It is at this point that community leaders decide whether or not a local hospital is required, how big it will be, and what services it will deliver. The desirable complement of physicians—their number and type—should also be determined during this stage. By building the system up from the population and its needs, the most delicate and most crucial decisions should rest on a firm base.

There is no way to avoid controversy in planning for health services. This is no reason to avoid the process. Local communities will be well served if they take planning into their own hands and make it a joint activity engaged in by the people who stand to benefit. Only by putting together an exact picture of the desired goal—in terms of bricks and mortar, people, and programs—can rural communities overcome a defensive posture. Health care arrangements in rural communities change over a period of 20–30 years as one generation of physicians retires and obsolete hospitals are replaced. Only by knowing what is desired in the next stage of development can a rural community be effective in seeing that its objectives are reached.

THE RURAL HEALTH SYSTEM SHOULD BE BASED ON GENERALISTS

The second principle revolves around the historically proven tenet that in the rural environment enterprises of all kinds are built on generalists. This necessity derives from the fundamental definition of rural living—a small, relatively remote population. Teachers, garage mechanics, lawyers, and health professionals all must have the capacity to operate effectively in a broad arena.

It is not merely chance that the fortunes of rural health services in America have fluctuated according to the relative supply and esteem of the general practitioner. The decline in the quality and quantity of rural health care paralleled the eclipse of the general practitioner. Smaller health care systems cannot depend primarily on specialists; this observation pertains for nurses, administrators, technicians, and dieticians, as well as physicians. Rural professionals must be comfortable with uncertainty, challenged by diversity, and flexible in their skills, working hours, and interpersonal style.

Those providing medical care are saddled with an additional burden not shared by other professionals. Since medical care must be available on a continuous basis, some system of coverage must be available for unscheduled problems. In fact, the unscheduled component of medical care is precisely the segment encompassing the most urgent and complex emergency problems. The mechanism used to deal with this uncertainty is the on-call system, in which health professionals in rotation maintain coverage during night, weekend, and holiday hours. Because there are few physicians and nurses in smaller communities, each individual must be willing and able to cover for a colleague along the entire breadth of medical practice. The narrowly trained specialist, although providing a valuable service to the community, is in general unwilling and unable to handle the potpourri of conditions that present at night, many of them potentially life threatening. Because the specialists cannot provide coverage for the generalists, nor the generalists for the specialists, all members of the medical community are forced to take on greater amounts of on-call obligation, which may undermine the stability of the entire system.

The same comments apply with equal weight to nursing and administrative staff. Nurses in rural hospitals are called upon to accept responsibility for obstetrics, new-born care, and intensive care, either sequentially or, at times, concurrently. Administrators must be able to deal with personnel, handle budgets, purchase a new refrigerator for the hospital kitchen, and manage a feisty group of county commissioners. In both instances, narrow educational experiences or highly developed technical skills in and of themselves are inadequate preparation for the rigors of the assignment. Competent, confident generalists must form the human foundation for the health care system at all levels.

Paradoxically, many educational and regulatory forces militate against production of the confident generalist. Within the health professions, two recent trends have impaired the ability of rural health care systems to find appropriately trained individuals. The first is specialization, a process of continually expanding the amount of time it takes and the amount of detail that must be mastered for a particular profession; the second is credentialing, as more and more groups within the health professional sphere seek independent professional status.

This trend is apparent, for example, in the field of nursing. There is a powerful push underway by academic leaders of the profession to require all registered nurses to complete a four-year baccalaureate degree in order to be eligible to work as nurses. Since the majority of all nurses in this country were not prepared through this route and most nursing schools do not grant the bachelor's degree, this proposal would cause major changes in the preparation of nurses. It would increase the length and expense of training, concentrate power in the hands of a relatively small number of educational institutions, and probably restrict the number of people obtaining nursing degrees.

The implications for rural areas are obvious. The supply of nurses would be more tenuous, the cost of nursing would increase, and the capacity and willingness of nurses to deal with the day-to-day nursing duties that make up the primary workload of the rural office or hospital would diminish. The same process has occurred in other areas, such as the preparation of laboratory and x-ray technicians, physical therapists, nutritionists, and other ancillary personnel.

Credentialing is a parallel phenomenon. As individual groups increase the length of their curricula and see themselves as professionals with specialized skills and a set of self-imposed standards, they desire the status and the financial rewards of autonomous, licensed professional groups. Respiratory therapists define a technological and patient care area and then attempt—through government recognition and regulation—to set barriers through exams and licensure to those who would practice in the field. The result may be an increase in quality, but a side-effect is an increase in the cost of health care and a decrease in administrative flexibility within the hospital. Small hospitals cannot afford to hire multiple ancillary specialists in increasingly narrow technical categories. In most cases the patient load is insufficient to fully occupy the time of the narrowly trained individual, and the efficiency of the hospital decreases as the costs and complexity rise.

The rural health care system needs generalists if it is to maintain resilience and stability. Specialized individuals and services may be added once the critical mass of generalists is maintained and the system is stable and in equilibrium. Rural administrators and representatives need to realize that they have a stake in assuring that generalists are being trained, licensed, and reimbursed by the local governmental authorities, and, thus, they must be active in the political and educational field. Rural community leaders should lend their political support to family practice programs and licensed practical nurse (LPN) training as one way of ensuring a future source of manpower.

ALL FUNCTIONS WITHIN A RURAL HEALTH CARE SYSTEM SHOULD BE INTEGRATED

Narrow, categorical programs have been of dubious benefit to rural health care. Although new services may be introduced into the area, the program may have side effects that cancel out its contribution. Each categorical program incurs administrative costs that ultimately must come from the funds designated for the target population. Rural programs, because of the small number of potential users and the large areas involved, are usually relatively costly, and often inefficient. Most disruptive is the tendency for the categorical program to siphon off clients who would otherwise use and support the basic health care system.

Most rural communities cannot generate enough demand to support multiple overlapping health care systems. All health care needs should be funneled, if possible, through the basic health care system, and duplication of services should be avoided. As we explored in the section on mental health care (Chapter 7), family physicians are the first recourse for most people with emotional difficulties. In a similar fashion, the local physicians and the hospital should be the focus of all other suitable services: rehabilitative care, physical therapy, laboratory and other diagnostic tests, and so forth. In this way, by channeling as much demand as possible through the basic system, the entire apparatus is strengthened professionally and economically.

Consolidation of services also reduces the amount of time and money that must go into administrative overhead. The same administrative staff and corporate structure that serve the local hospital can accept the sponsorship and handle the paperwork for a home health care or chore worker service. At the same time, incorporating additional services under the umbrella of the hospital increases the revenue for that institution, improves the penetration of the hospital into the local market, and spreads administrative costs over a broader base of activities.

This principle is in many ways a corollary of the generalist concept. Rural communities cannot afford the luxury of multiple single-purpose programs, all competing for the same limited number of clients, wrestling with the problem of recruiting urban-trained professionals, and then facing insurmountable difficulties in creating sufficient demand or solving transportation problems. Rural communities must pull together rather than allow themselves to be pulled apart.

RURAL COMMUNITIES MUST BUILD TWO-WAY COOPERATIVE ARRANGEMENTS WITH OTHER RURAL AND URBAN COMMUNITIES

Many rural areas display an apparent paranoia about working cooperatively with other communities. Part of this fear is justifiable;

part is illogical. No single community is entirely self-sufficient with regard to health services. There are always some services that are so rarely done or are so complex that only a few centers in the world perform them. The smaller the population base of the medical service area, the greater the number of services that must be sought outside the community. It is very much in the rural community's interest to enter into cooperative arrangements with other areas to assure that these services will be predictably available in a time of need.

It is perhaps more typical of most rural communities to resist cooperative arrangements, spurred by the fear they will be swallowed up by the larger institutions with which they work. There is a tendency on the part of regional centers to act as great vortexes that pull patients to them and retain them as long as possible, thus undermining the rural health care systems of the communities where these patients originate. However, it is only by establishing a firm agreement ahead of time that rural areas can resist this powerful centripetal force. There is a quid pro quo—professional and economic—operating powerfully in the health field, and it is this mutuality of interest that can benefit both sides in a cooperative agreement.

Rural areas by their nature and inclination concentrate on primary health care services, both in the ambulatory and inpatient realm. Regional centers and urban areas provide some primary services but tend to base their identity on the specialized tasks which they perform. Most rural physicians and hospitals can choose among several alternative locations when referring patients. Most regional centers compete actively for patients and are willing to extend themselves to secure a steady stream of patient referrals from peripheral sources. This mutual self-interest must be the basis of cooperative agreements.

Cooperative arrangements take many forms; we have described a wide variety of them earlier in Chapter 6. No matter what the form, certain aspects of agreements should be constant. Rural communities should ensure that patients are returned to their home communities when they no longer require the specialized services of the referral center. The cooperating urban institution must perform a spectrum of outreach services to help the rural community maintain its standards of care. These include ready consultation and actual visits to the smaller community for on-site assistance and continuing education. The agreement must in fact benefit both parties without undermining either.

Most rural areas have many ad hoc cooperative arrangements in place. Physicians for the most part develop referral networks based on their experience in training and practice. Physicians are much more comfortable referring patients to people whom they know and respect; for this reason circuit-riding courses by hospitals and medical schools are an excellent source of patient referrals. However, frequently rural communities reap only a fraction of the potential benefits that could be extracted from the referral relationship. Nursing and administrative consultation are just as valuable to the rural system, but rarely do rural communities effectively use their bargaining clout in securing a comprehensive cooperative relationship.

The growing number and success of the proprietary hospital chains demonstrate the utility of formalized cooperative arrangements. By drawing on a much richer network of resources, rural hospitals can similarly improve their performance, decrease their isolation, and build—not diminish—their patient volume. The key is that rural leaders must be deliberate in the way they enter into such agreements and realize that they have considerable latitude in the types of arrangements they foster. Rural communities need to work together in building these sensitive and sensible regional networks, rather than dissipate their energies competing fruitlessly with each other.

THE STRUCTURE OF THE REIMBURSEMENT SYSTEM MUST REWARD APPROPRIATE RURAL HEALTH SERVICES

The market for health services is largely shaped by those who pay the bills. The majority of health care costs are shunted through third-party payers, government agencies, insurance companies, and associations that buffer consumers from the cost of the health care they use. This has the advantage of increasing the number of people with access to health care services and mitigating the financial impact of illness. It has the disadvantage of insulating the consumer from the fiscal consequence of unnecessary utilization and thus increasing the cost of health care. By paying more for some services than others, third-party payers shape and distort the health care market.

This last effect is particularly pernicious in rural areas. Third-party payers tend to reimburse most readily and most generously those who perform quantifiable services; surgery is an excellent example. It is easy to recognize and count an appendectomy, and the surgeon who performs the service is well rewarded for his or her operative tour de force. It is difficult to recognize or count a visit for health education or counseling. Insurance schemes pay poorly if at all for these services.

Third-party payers do not set policy; they follow prevailing customs. In medicine, they tend to enshrine and reinforce the disparities that exist between the money flowing to urban versus rural areas. Urban physicians tend to charge more for an office visit; therefore Medicare pays them more for an office visit. Urban specialists dominate the Blue Cross and Blue Shield boards that set insurance premiums and the benefit structure; technical procedures are rewarded much more handsomely than straightforward diagnosis and treatment. Counseling, health promotion, and prevention usually are not paid for at all. The net effect is to drain money from rural areas in the form of taxes and premiums that are only partially returned. The cycle is reinforcing. Lower fees lead to lower salaries and less capability to attract and retain health personnel of all types.

This situation will be one of the most difficult to change yet is of crucial importance. It is an area in which policy formulation and control lie outside the rural community.

THERE ARE THRESHOLDS IN RURAL HEALTH CARE; CERTAIN LEVELS OF SERVICE REQUIRE EXTERNAL SUBSIDY

Health services are hierarchical in nature. Everyone requires certain basic services, such as immunization. Most people use and benefit from outpatient medical services for minor illnesses. The majority of people will at some time be patients in a hospital, having babies, getting their bones set or their pneumonia treated. Fewer people will ever be in a nursing home, but most will have family members who at some point will use such an institution. Only a small fraction of the population will have open-heart surgery. One in a million will have a bone marrow transplant.

Which services should be available in rural communities? The first principle suggests that this can be determined by knowing the size and composition of the population served and applying considerations of cost and quality as yardsticks in making the decision. Yet there are many very small rural communities where the aggregate demand is insufficient to support any permanent health care system.

As we discussed in Chapter 4, it is highly unlikely that areas with fewer than 4,000 people will support physicians; areas with fewer than 1,500 people will have difficulty maintaining a midlevel practitioner. These are relative population thresholds that impose certain economic restrictions on the scope of services that can be maintained given our current medical care marketplace. However, the marketplace alone should not be the ultimate arbiter of the way in which medical services are distributed.

It is to society's benefit that certain services be available to all. Immunization is an example in which the ultimate beneficiary may not be the person receiving the inoculation but those who are thus protected from exposure to the disease. By the same token, it is to society's benefit to continue to support small, dispersed communities, in order to maintain social heterogeneity and cultural richness. In order to maintain this diversity, certain health services must be available to the people who live in these smaller communities. Below certain population thresholds, maintenance of these services will require explicit external subsidy.

Many of the rural health programs that were spawned in the 1970s will never attain self-sufficiency. Certain areas will require support to maintain even the most rudimentary health station. Small rural areas should realize this and not become frustrated at their seeming inferiority in not being able to totally support the level of health services they feel are essential. In order to maintain equity in the receipt of health services, there needs to be an appreciation that certain areas will never be able to totally defray their own costs. Federal and state governments have a responsibility to identify and support basic health programs in these areas.

APPLYING THE PRINCIPLES TO SPECIFIC ASPECTS OF THE RURAL HEALTH CARE SYSTEM

In earlier chapters we have set out an approach toward providing the key health services required by rural communities. The following section selects four important aspects of the rural health care system for the purpose of emphasis, using the six principles in an attempt to further illuminate solutions to persistent problems in the delivery of rural health care services.

THE RURAL HOSPITAL

The rural hospital is the center of the rural health care system. Although it is possible to build an adequate health care system in a community without a hospital, our current mode of delivering health care depends heavily on the hospital for a broad range of important services. The hospital is an extension of the community and relatively independent of the personalities of the health care providers. The presence of the hospital means that the machinery that is needed to deliver services, hire physicians, raise money, and receive reimbursement is intact. It is not chance that rural communities hold onto their hospitals with ferocious tenacity.

The rural hospital is also one of the weak links in the system. In Chapter 6 we explored the problems with cost and quality that plague many rural hospitals. The community must be willing to take an entirely dispassionate look at its hospital, catalogue its failings, and develop a plan to shore up and improve the facility. The worst possible approach is to wait until falling occupancy rates, a failed hospital levy, or severe deficiencies noted on the state's annual inspection force the hospital over the brink. Many rural communities have gone from crisis to crisis, patching up one deficiency after another without at any time achieving any fundamental improvement in the function of the hospital. Too frequently the hospital fails despite these attempts at repair, and the money invested in rear-guard actions is unrecoverable.

Perhaps one of the most disruptive situations occurs when the community is held hostage by one or several physicians who continually threaten to leave town if their dictates are ignored. The threat paralyzes the hospital board and town leaders, who are afraid they will lose everything if they antagonize their physicians. Unless the community calls the physicians' bluffs, and takes some responsibility for the type of health care that will be delivered, the situation invariably produces more problems than could ever be generated by the physicians' departures. New physicians are excluded from the town or driven out soon after arrival. The hospital tends to degenerate or become involved in activities of questionable propriety or safety. And the health care system is static, unable to change or respond to new conditions.

The only workable recourse is for the community leaders to develop a systematic plan for their community's health system and then work patiently and slowly to bring it about. If there is a strong and unified community base, it is possible to create a setting that will be attractive to new physicians. Older, recalcitrant physicians can be circumvented, coerced, or occasionally even convinced to become more pliant. Failing hospitals can be redesigned to provide more appropriate care and to attract a larger portion of the population.

As noted previously, rural hospitals can diversify, using their plant and administrative machinery to serve many purposes not necessarily related to inpatient care. Cooperative arrangements must be forged with other hospitals. Physician consultants can often be coaxed to rotate periodically through the community, the cost of the services totally defrayed through patient care services and the generation of referrals. Government agencies will often extend themselves to help threatened rural hospitals, particularly if the political process is used to help get their attention. The key to all these activities is to know where the community wishes to go in health care and to realize that the basis for a revitalized hospital is broad local community support.

BUILDING STRONG PHYSICIAN PRACTICES

Doctors are essential to an adequate rural health care system. Even in small towns staffed by midlevel practitioners, the longevity of the provider, the quality of care, and the acceptability of the practice will depend upon some alliance with a cooperating physician. In most rural communities, physicians will be at the center of the health care system.

Rural communities should be actively involved in assuring the proper mix of physicians for their town. Physicians differ greatly in their training, skill, orientation, and compatibility. Too frequently, physician recruitment is exclusively within the doctor's province; it should be a shared responsibility. Physicians are not necessarily the best judges of the needs of the community and often are swayed by economic or personality considerations when asked to determine what additional physicians should be invited to practice. On the other hand, town leaders should be sensitive to the local physicians' preferences and attempt to recruit new doctors who will be compatible with the current staff and also build the overall strength of the health care system.

One attractive option for rural communities is to base their health care system on residency-trained family practitioners. Recently trained family doctors have the breadth of skill and the depth of training to function in a small community and practice at a level that earns them the respect and collaboration of other specialists. One recruiting technique is to make contact with existing regional family practice training programs and entice the residents to rural communities to sample the life style and test the waters of medical practice. Other specialties can complement those in general practice, but the foundation should be secure before too much effort is devoted to attracting more narrowly trained professionals.

For most rural communities, a three-to-four-person family practice group should be the first objective in building a strong local physician practice. Once this nucleus has been created, it will in most cases be self-replicating. If individual partners leave, they can be readily replaced. No matter which specialists are or are not available within the local area, the local physician group can assure the provision of basic primary and hospital care. Until this nucleus is in place, the system is unstable. Multispecialty group practices are another option but usually are suitable only in larger rural communities.

With the family practice group as the foundation, the community can then begin the process of adding additional talents. Many of these can be provided by itinerant visiting specialists as described earlier. These arrangements should for the most part be made with and through the local physicians, although the hospital can provide space and staff support. Radiology, pathology, and various sub-specialties of internal medicine and surgery are best provided initially through the itinerant approach. Some of these physicians may well choose to locate permanently in the community as a result of the exposure.

Additional specialists can be added as part of the long-range planning for the community's health services. A general surgeon, a pediatrician, and a general internist are examples of the types of specialists who complement the existing family medicine group. It is important to work closely with the local physicians to work out a suitable work arrangement; sometimes the specialists will join the existing group. More frequently they will work independently.

In certain communities it may be necessary to subsidize practices during the start-up phase. If medical practice has deteriorated in a town, it usually requires several years to rebuild the previous base of public support and usage. It is very common for there to be some physician turnover during this phase until the right chemistry is achieved between town and doctor. Subsidizing the physician by guaranteeing salaries or defraying a portion of overhead expenses is a good investment for the local community.

Communities do not have the luxury of remaining ignorant about the intricacies of medical practice. Unless they understand the tribulations and the rewards of country practice, they will be unable to attract and retain people with the spectrum of skills that rural areas require. Community leaders must also become active in that part of the political process that makes decisions about the number and type of physicians to be trained within the state. With federal involvement in medical education diminishing rapidly, state governments will play an increasingly important role. Primary care specialties like family medicine have difficulty supporting extensive training programs without earmarked governmental support. It is in the interest of rural communities to ensure that such support is maintained.

Physicians occupy an unusual spot in the social structure of rural communities. From an economic standpoint, they are successful entrepreneurs, well-paid business people similar to bankers and lawyers. On the other hand, they are also social servants like policemen or teachers, just as essential to the welfare and functioning of the community but paid for through a fee-for-service mechanism outside of local community control. This anomalous status requires some fairly innovative interpersonal and structural relationships to strike a workable balance. Health care is too important an area to be left entirely to physicians.

FOSTERING MEANINGFUL COMMUNITY INVOLVEMENT

Building a health care system is a community endeavor. The community has two crucial roles to play. First, it must participate in the design, implementation, and sustenance of the system. Secondly, in rural areas particularly, members of the community must be involved as volunteers in the provision of medical care in areas such as emergency services.

Health care planning is a local responsibility. If local communities want to have the kind of health services that fit their needs, they must be intimately involved in shaping the system. Health care politics at the local level can provide an opportunity for modeling community cooperation, or it can degenerate into divisive shouting matches between feuding factions. In many communities the hospital board, which usually ends up as the most important health institution in the community, is not considered a desirable assignment. Yet the community must ensure that its true leaders play a part at this level for the system to work. Membership on the hospital board should be a coveted assignment, and local government must remain informed about and supportive of health care programs.

Participation should be as broad as possible. Community associations to which people make contributions by way of dues are excellent vehicles for creating a feeling of ownership among the populace. Health fairs, fund-raising drives, open houses, newspaper stories, and elections for members of various health-related community boards also build a strong base of support. Since the ultimate success of the rural health care system depends on its being utilized by the local population, these activities also serve an important public relations function. If people play a part in building their health care system, they are more likely to trust it and turn to it in time of need.

In addition, rural health care systems depend on volunteers to deliver critical health services. The emergency medical care system is vital to the community, not only in potentially saving lives by improving the rapidity and adequacy of response to emergencies, but also by giving people some feeling of security. The emergency medical services (EMS) system depends upon volunteer labor and requires that ordinary people become relatively sophisticated in one domain of medical practice. The EMS system also serves to weld together the community, to create enormous pride and esprit de corps among those who are active participants, and to increase the general level of medical sophistication.

As we discussed in Chapter 7, reliance on community volunteers can also greatly improve mental health services in rural communities. Other health services can also be handled expeditiously by volunteers; home visiting programs, work in the hospital and nursing home auxiliaries, and participation in health planning bodies all strengthen the local health system at the same time they increase local involvement. The objective of all these efforts is to improve the scope and quality of local services and foster a feeling of community ownership in the local health care system.

MAKING GOVERNMENT A HELPFUL PARTNER IN RURAL HEALTH CARE

Government intervention in the health field has had a tremendous impact in the last few decades. The new social programs created during the 1970s have, for the most part, had a salutary effect on the ability of rural communities to obtain health services. We have discussed these programs in detail. The challenge for the rest of this century is to maintain the best elements of the structures created by these programs and to learn to apply the lessons that we have learned as part of this widespread social experiment.

Government in the United States is not monolithic. It is an extremely malleable and multifaceted entity, exquisitely sensitive to political pressures and mercurial social forces. Part of the problem with the programs of the 1970s was that in many ways they were contradictory, fighting themselves. This is particularly true in the health care field.

Many of the categorical programs had major rural health components: the National Health Service Corps, Migrant Health Act, Community Mental Health Centers, and on and on. Each of these programs made a contribution in some way, even though many times the contributions were fragmentary, poorly coordinated, ill conceived, or poorly managed. However, they did make a contribution by increasing the amount of resources targeted at inhabitants of rural areas.

During the same period, other government activities, such as health planning laws, Medicare reimbursement policies, hospital licensing criteria, and increased credentialing, have had a negative impact on rural areas. The bureaucratic obstacles become more ponderous and more complex, the requirements more stringent, and the entire delivery system more distorted as the result of reimbursement policies that reward technologically intensive care at the expense of primary care. All these programs grew out of a commitment to improve access to health care, but at no point in the federal or state structure was there any coordinated policy for rural health care. The programmatic collisions were side effects of well-intentioned laws and actions, but in many cases one program would inadvertently nullify the effects of another program.

The coming decades will see a severe pruning of the federal tree. Many programs will be discarded, and, unfortunately, there appears to be little attempt to make a distinction among the programs on the basis of relative value. The following guidelines would make government a steadier and more effective partner in the attempt to improve rural health care. They may or may not be achievable in the present political climate, but they offer some direction to rural individuals trying to influence the political process.

Develop Policies Specific to Rural Areas.   Rural areas have a different set of problems than urban areas. Policies that do not distinguish between rural and urban problems injure rural areas by forcing them to comply with standards that confer little benefit. It would be useful to develop a regulatory framework specific to rural America and its needs.

Transform the Reimbursement System to Reward Basic Primary Care.   This perhaps quixotic goal is crucial to the improvement of the entire medical care system. We currently reward indiscriminately every technological advance, no matter how costly or unproven, while we often do not pay anything for basic health services of proven value. Until the economic system gives a different signal to the providers of medical care and technology, the complexity and cost of care will continue to escalate. Rural areas cannot, and should not, compete in the technological arena. They have a major stake in a revised reimbursement system.

Build a Mechanism for Long-Term Planning into the Governmental System.   Planning has been totally discredited in the minds of most rural dwellers. If a system is to replace the current one, it must be more stable centrally, prevent dizzying swings in federal policy, and allow for increased local responsibility. Federal programs are buffeted by political winds to the degree that rural inhabitants fear participation because the future is always so murky. We should experiment with the novel idea of setting a course and sticking to it, allowing some consistency and predictability in federal programming.

These concepts are probably of little immediate practical utility. Our political system is volatile by its nature; its great strength and great weakness are its responsiveness to political expressions. We are currently entering a period of austerity and retrenchment, the product of ideological belief and economic necessity. The pendulum will reach the end of its excursion and begin its predictable arc back toward an era of renewed government interest in social welfare and equity. During the interim, rural communities must build upon the advances of the previous 10 years in health care and seek to modify those portions of the program that have inhibited rather than enhanced the building of stronger health care systems.

Focus Efforts at the State and Regional Level.   As the federal government withdraws from its active role in the delivery of rural health services, one excellent and logical recourse is the states themselves. States have played an increasingly important role in this field over the last decade. Some of the earliest and most far-reaching programs have been developed at the state level, largely in response to the shortage of rural physicians that became so apparent in the 1960s and 1970s. A second stimulus behind state involvement was the often confusing array of federal programs with narrow categorical objectives that pertained to rural areas, leading states to establish organizational clearinghouses through which the programs could be coordinated. The result of both these forces has been the creation of an institutional focus in many states that is responsible for rural health programs and problems.

Perhaps the broadest state effort is that of the Office of Rural Health Services in North Carolina. This component of the North Carolina Department of Health Resources is involved in almost every aspect of rural health, including basic research, community development, construction of health facilities, training of health providers, recruitment of physicians and other health workers, and continuing medical education. This office has served as the funnel through which federal resources are deployed to individual communities and has greatly improved the distribution of health care and the integration of the rural health care system. The effort in North Carolina, while quite sophisticated and well funded, can be readily duplicated and should be encouraged in other parts of the country. The fact that many states have adopted some variation on this theme attests to the political feasibility of this kind of effort.

PROSPECTS AND IMPLICATIONS FOR THE FUTURE

Health care is a reflection of current social beliefs and values. The status of health care services in rural areas depends upon the relative vitality of that segment of our society as well as our current concept of health and disease.

Rural life is undergoing a resurgence, a resurgence that will probably be sustained by emerging decentralization in our society. Large urban centers are rapidly losing population, and, despite increased energy costs, many people are choosing to live in rural areas. The advent of the age of the microcomputer and satellite transmission has allowed industrial decentralization at a time when personal preference makes it possible to attract workers to rural settings. Rapid growth in the extractive industries has also created a shift in the work force to sparsely populated areas. In the wake of these population shifts will come a clamor for more stable and more sophisticated health care services.

The health care complex is reaching an impasse. The impasse is largely fiscal. Our capacity to create new diagnostic and therapeutic modalities has outstripped our ability to pay for them. Escalation in health care costs cannot continue at the current rate for the simple mathematical reason that at some point in the near future there will no longer be enough money to pay for all the services we know how to produce. Medical care costs have already begun to deplete our capacity to pay for other desirable social services, such as education and environmental protection.

This zero sum game has been obscured by the way we organize, deliver, and buy medical services, but this sleight of hand cannot be sustained indefinitely. When the collision comes, we will be forced to make specific choices between painful alternatives. What technology do we want to pay for? What is the impact of increasingly sophisticated medical services on the quality of individual and collective human life?

It is our feeling that rural areas will benefit from this self-examination. Rural communities already face, and must solve, the problems of reconciling finite resources with infinitely beguiling technologies. Because of limited demand for certain costly services, rural hospitals deliberately do not add them to their clinical repertoire. Each additional health care component must pass some test of rationality—at least implicitly—before it is added to the existing menu. Because rural communities have experience in such judgments and because they generally are not encumbered with expensive and questionable technologies, they will be less affected by the growing fiscal crisis.

In fact, the rural health care delivery system may serve as an example for other segments of the society struggling with the tradeoffs between paying for ever more costly medical care and retaining flexibility to support other social services. The conflict will revolve around emotionally charged issues and will ultimately be solved through some sort of external constraint. Government agencies at the federal or state level may place explicit ceilings on the number of specialists allowed to practice in various areas. Certain classes of procedures, such as heart transplants, may be eliminated as benefits under health insurance schemes. If rural areas are able to use defensible planning standards as a guide to shaping rational systems of care, the solutions they evolve may be adopted by urban areas where conflict resolution is more difficult.

Rural health care also has the potential to lead the way in humanizing medical care, in combatting the alienation and dependence that our current medical care ethos tends to perpetuate. Because rural health care providers are manifestly members of the communities they serve and because rural health care systems depend on community participation and volunteer labor to function, health is repatriated. There is a widespread and deeply felt revulsion against the depersonalization engendered by modern medical care, a revulsion expressed in ways as divergent as home births and megavitamin therapy. This growing breach between the public and the profession can be bridged in rural areas. This experience may spill over into other educational and practice institutions and improve the system for all.

The last two decades have been exciting and productive ones for the field of rural health care. There has been a basic realization that rural areas have significant difficulty in obtaining decent health care, and many of the educational and programmatic innovations have been rapidly translated into more and better health care in rural America. Despite a contracting government role in the areas of health and social welfare, we expect the momentum generated to continue to have an effect. This coupled with a basic renaissance in rural society, should help to make the coming decades productive ones for rural areas.

Index